THE COST of

BEING SICK

BY NICHOLAS J. WEBB

Published by:

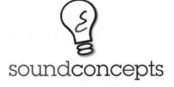

soundconcepts

Sound Concepts, Inc.
15 East 400 South
Orem, Utah 84058

800.544.7044

www.soundconcepts.com

ISBN   1-887938-97-4

I would like to dedicate this book to my

beautiful wife, Michelle, my daughters

Taylor and Madison, and my son, Chase.

I would also like to thank Colby Allen,

Colby Olds, Dr. Peggy Gardner, Dr. Paul

Davis, Brian O' Connell, Dr. Mitchell

Akman, and Curtis Freeman.

Nicholas J. Webb

Table of Contents

Foreword

Through administrative roles in medical education, research, and managing outpatient clinics in a large non-profit hospital, I have experienced firsthand this impending health-care "crisis." The impact of healthful behaviors cannot be oversimplified. I have observed the shock and sense of helplessness of patients' families in the face of illness. At the same time, I have watched patients tethered to IV poles smoking in outside "provided" areas. The health crisis we face has a curious tendency to invert itself.

Nick Webb is fully aware of the importance of research and development. He recognizes that continued training and education of medical health staff is the foundation of excellent medicine. As an owner, manager, and entrepreneur in the medical device field, Nick understands that American medicine is a costly enterprise. But in this book he issues a proclamation that major governmental, institutional, and personal rehabilitation must occur if we are to emerge from this crisis as a healthy and health-giving nation.

The underlying theme of this book is not a novel moral philosophy—it is a simple response to the health-care crisis: examine the issues, take care of yourself, and help others. Take the national rise in emergency room visits, higher acuity of inpatients, and demands for new technology in the face of reduced resources and reimbursement, and it is clear that the government's health system provides little or no incentive for practitioners or their patients to help them look after themselves.

The current economics of medicine will not foster change. The codified reimbursement system is based on an illness model. With only 2 percent of its health-care budget focused on prevention, a track record of failed HMOs trying to ratchet down escalating costs by rationing resources in the name of "health maintenance," and more than forty million of its people uninsured, American health care is in a downward spiral of exploding costs. The obvious alternative supports cost containment measures that may be contrary to the moral underpinnings of our society.

We prize the evolutionary advances of medicine in imaging, minimally invasive surgeries, and designer drugs. But perhaps this evolution obscures a hard truth—the devolution of the health status of Americans. We are justifiably proud of a medical model that eases disease, blocks pain, and sometimes cures the incurable. Although grounded in the code of Hippocrates, American medicine is driven by economic forces beyond the control of the "system" itself and always subject to the siren call of new technology.

Nick Webb's argument is not in contradiction to the awesome enterprise of American medicine. His argument speaks to the necessity of social progress toward good personal health and demands that we restore some sound principles of good health to the way we live our lives and influence our children to live theirs.

Dr. Peggy Gardner

Introduction

In his 1961 farewell address, President Dwight D. Eisenhower coined the term "military-industrial complex." According to *The Longman Guide to World Affairs*, Eisenhower warned the American people to not permit their most important national decisions to be influenced by the narrow, special interests of a large military and the defense industries that support it.

More than forty years later Eisenhower's words might well have read:

> This conjunction of an immense medical establishment and a large pharmaceutical industry is new in the American experience. The total influence—economic, political and even spiritual—is felt in every city, every statehouse and every office of the federal government. We recognize the imperative need for this development. Yet we must not fail to comprehend its grave implications. Our toil, resources and livelihood are all involved—so is the very structure of our society.

> In the councils of government, we must guard against the acquisition of unwarranted influence, whether sought or unsought, by the medical-industrial complex. The potential for the disastrous rise of misplaced power exists and will persist.

> We must never let the weight of this combina-
> tion endanger our liberties or democratic
> processes. We should take nothing for granted.
> Only an alert and knowledgeable citizenry can
> compel the proper meshing of the huge indus-
> trial and medical machinery of treatment with
> our healthy lifestyles and goals so that well-
> being and liberty may prosper together.

While Eisenhower actually cautioned against the military-industrial complex, his words also hold true as an alert for the American citizenry regarding the growing influence of the medical-industrial complex. Though the term is not unique to me, medical-industrial complex is an appropriate description for what we are seeing today. The medical-industrial complex is made up of the FDA, which dictates the types of treatments via approvals; doctors and hospitals that deliver treatments based on reimbursement; and governments and insurance companies, which authorize and thus control reimbursements.

Due to advances in technology, biotechnology, and medicine that were designed to produce healthier lifestyles and longer lives, Americans are adapting way too easily to unhealthy lifestyles in full confidence that if they do get sick there's a miracle pill a phone call away that will cure what ails them. It's a mindset that the medical-industrial complex is only too happy to accommodate. After all, they enter our homes with comforting television commercials that show the next gen-eration of "perfect little pills" that will make all the aches and pains go away—at least until it's time to take the next dose.

But the damage being done by the conventional wisdom that prescription drugs are the best answer to our health-care problems is catastrophic. According to a recent study by RAND on the ill effects of our fast food, super-sized lifestyles, the way we live is directly attributable to the skyrocketing costs of health care. The study reported that obesity is associated with a 36 percent increase in inpatient and outpatient expenditures and a 77 percent increase in medication. The study reinforced growing concerns about how dramatically increasing rates of obesity in the U.S. will negatively affect health-care costs as well as overall public health.

But what's being done to prevent obesity? Not much.

Consider the insidious impact of heart disease, a highly preventable ailment that continues to grow unchecked in America today. According to the U.S. Center for Disease Control and Prevention (CDC), heart disease remains the leading cause of death in the United States despite better health care and more public awareness of the dangers of smoking, inactivity, and poor diet. "We're still a sedentary society. We still eat foods that are high in calories and high in fat. We still smoke a lot. A lot of Americans have not gotten their high blood pressure under control," said Janice Williams of the CDC's National Center for Chronic Disease Prevention and Health Promotion.

Thus heart disease remains the leading killer of American men and women even though most Americans are well aware of the dangers of the disease after four decades of public information on the topic. One reason for this seeming indifference is that the medical-industrial complex has convinced many Americans that treatment for heart disease is readily available instead of emphasizing that preventive measures to thwart heart disease before it occurs are also readily available. The CDC noted that during the 1990s "there was minimal, if any, improvement" in behaviors that have been linked to heart ailments.

At $10 a pop for some temporary relief from the symptoms fueled by our super-sized lifestyles, who's going to complain? Not the grateful masses, whose employers pay exorbitant amounts for prescription benefits plans. Not the beleaguered, litigation-shy doctors who prescribe those prescriptions. And certainly not the pharmaceutical firms that, in the fine tradition of Scrooge McDuck, spend their days wallowing in the billions of dollars they've made by selling those prescriptions.

Who's going to blow the whistle on such a lucrative racket?

I am.

My name is Nicholas Webb, and I've spent a lifetime studying the medical-industrial complex and its debilitating effects on the American health-care system. As chief executive officer at several successful health-care companies, advisor to hospitals and medical research organizations, and the recipient of twenty-seven patents from the U.S. Patent and Trademark Office for medical inventions, I've learned a thing or two about the way our health-care system is structured—and how it's cataclysmic breakdown is inevitable unless we take drastic action.

That's where this book helps. Through *The Cost of Being Sick*, I'm going to show you how our lifestyles, the medical-industrial complex, and our health-care system have converged to the critical point where they're actually working against us. They're doing so by focusing our health-care efforts on post-disease pills rather than prevention and on treating illness rather than promoting wellness. Up until now, the health-care industry has gotten away with it—with the tacit approval of that same American public that is too stressed-out and super-sized to put up much of a fight.

I know—harsh.

In writing this book, I realize I'm tackling some sacred cows that don't want you to think differently about your health care. That's why this book is one that the medical-industrial complex doesn't want you to read. Anything that suggests that our cure-now-worry-about-prevention-later health-care mentality has finally caught up with us is anathema to the folks who've lined their pockets with the profits they've made from billions of dollars in prescription drugs.

In *The Cost of Being Sick*, I'll show you how much money is being wasted on the treatment side of health care, and how much money—and how many lives—can be saved by turning the industry upside down and focusing on the preventive side of the health-care equation. I'll show you why "wellness" will be the watchword for health care in the 2000s.

Here's my promise to you: By the time you finish reading *The Cost of Being Sick*, I guarantee that you will never look at health care the same way again, and that you'll develop a new mindset on how to live your life in a healthy, happy manner, free of the treatment-based tyranny of the medical-industrial complex.

It won't be easy. It's never easy looking at old traditions in new ways. But when those traditions begin breaking down and threatening our culture, what other choice do we have?

For Americans, the clock is ticking. Consequently, creating new ways to look at health care at this late hour isn't a luxury—it's a necessity.

Chapter One

Future America
The Good, the Bad and the Ugly!

In the mid '90s, when my wife and I were expecting our daughter, Taylor, the media brought to light the unimaginable occurrence of infants going home from the hospital with the wrong set of parents. I began researching this problem and found one organization that estimated that every hour nearly three babies were accidentally switched. That was sixty-four babies a day—or 20,000 in a year—that were given to the wrong parents. We had never heard about these switches because the majority of time the switches were corrected before discharging. But that was not necessarily the problem. The real concern was the possibility of cross-contamination. During the time babies were with the wrong mother, they could have been exposed to any number of communicable diseases including herpes, HIV, or AIDS.

This isn't to say that our obstetric system was faulty, or that incompetent professionals were running it. The problem lay in the process of matching mother to child. The most common system practiced in hospitals was to put identically numbered bands on both the mother and infant. In my eyes, the possibility of mismatching numbers in the nursery was just too great!

I wasn't willing to take a chance of this happening with my wife and child. Subsequently, I developed a new banding system that utilizes a hand-held computer to scan both the mother and the baby. "KidMatch"—as the product was named—links mother to child through technology to help insure safety for both mom and baby. A correct match plays the tune of a familiar lullaby, while incorrect matches are signaled by an audible alarm. Not long after, hospital nurseries around the country adopted KidMatch.

Similarly, in today's magazines and newspapers a similar health tragedy is unfolding. Presidential, senatorial, and local government races are being influenced by the precarious state of government-funded health-care initiatives and the movement within corporate America to shift the burden of rising health insurance coverage to a more equal footing with its employees.

Thirty years ago this same system could easily handle treatment costs. At that time, the expense of administering these services to constituents and employees did not include the escalating price of treating our nation's three big killers. As the rate of incidence and cost of treating cancer, heart disease and diabetes continues to escalate, so too does the expense required by the government and corporate America.

The challenge lawmakers and executive committees face is whether they can justify to their voters and shareholders coverage for illnesses that are predominantly driven by poor lifestyle habits. Take cancer for example. According to the Harvard Medical School, only 30 percent of cancers are genetic in origin. The other 70 percent are directly related to lifestyle choices. If we take out tobacco-related cancers— which make up about 30 percent of cancers—we are left with 40 percent of all cancers being related to diet and exercise. Employers cannot be held financially responsible for the gradual health risks associated with frequent drive-thru lunches and super-sized meal deals.

Yet, on the flip side, employees are justifiably weary of benefit cuts when the media has shed new light on corporate greed, accounting shenanigans, and outrageous golden parachutes. Each side of this argument can easily find reasons to point a finger. Nevertheless, the solution to this divisive issue is not the capitulation of either side but the simple acceptance of responsibility.

The U.S. health-care system is perched on a cliff awaiting a tipping point where it will fall to an unfortunate demise. The only way to avoid the toppling of the system is to encourage prevention and wellness themes and de-emphasize treatment-based health-care initiatives. In the coming years we will see changes in the health-care industry that will impact you, the consumer, in significant ways. For more than two decades I have been involved in the solution side of medicine. I have provided tools and devices for a number of problems, yet these trends are leading to changes that no tool or device can fix. In the near future, we will see the impending crisis bare its teeth in the form of the following seven predictions:

1. Our Top Three Killers Will Grow Even More Lethal.

The danger of our poor diets and emphasis on treatment over prevention will result in a catastrophic rise in the number of cancer cases in the next 15 years. Health industry estimates peg the total number of cancer cases by 2020 at 15 million—about 50 percent more than we have today. And tomorrow's cancer will no longer be a condition associated with aging. Just as type II diabetes (formally known as adult on-set diabetes) is now an epidemic with our children, cancer will prey indiscriminately on people of all ages. The youth of thousands will inevitably be interrupted with trips to the hospital for chemo and radiation therapies.

Currently, diabetes is ranked as the sixth highest cause of death among Americans. In 1999, 68,399 people died from diabetes, while an additional 141,265 listed diabetes as a contributing factor to death. In the near future, you can count on that number rising as well as diabetes ranking as a cause of death. Currently, seventeen million people have diabetes—151,000 of which are under the age of twenty. According to the American Diabetes Association, the occurrence of type II diabetes is becoming more and more common, especially among children and adolescents. Diabetics have two times the risk of death compared to non-diabetics. And that's not to mention the common side effects of diabetes, which include heart disease, stroke, blindness, kidney disease, nervous system disease, dental disease, pregnancy complications, and amputation.

You can't talk about causes of death in America without talking about cardiovascular disease. Heart attacks and stroke account for the first and third rankings in causes of death. The leading cause of heart disease is largely a lifestyle factor. Atherosclerosis, or hardening of the arteries, is caused by a buildup of plaque in the blood vessels. This buildup leads to high blood pressure, weakened blood vessels and clogged arteries. Our diet—which is predominantly high in fat—and lack of exercise are significant contributors to this problem. And it's not just adults who are suffering from this disease. The June 2000 *Harvard Health Letter* surprised many with the indication that atherosclerosis can begin as early as age nine.

2. Employees Will Bear the Burden of Health-Care Costs.

This is less a prediction and more inevitability. Health-care costs are rising at almost 15 percent annually, according to the Kaiser Family Foundation. That fact is virtually choking small businesses, which employ about half of all workers in America. The National Federation of Independent Business recently concluded a four-month study that isolated insurance as the No. 1 problem for small business. Unable to cope with such increases, businesses will pass along the escalating costs of health care to employees. According to a March 3, 2003, article in *Fortune* magazine, "Health care, in fact, has become what hours and wages and job security were in the past—the make-or-break issue upon which unions and employers are increasingly giving no quarter." Medical costs will rise. Companies will protect profits. Employees will ultimately feel the squeeze on their paychecks.

3. Health-Care Costs Will Become the "New" Mortgage.

Imagine monthly health-care bills of more than $1,000 per month, or paying out $12,000 per year for health care on a salary of $40,000. That's where we are heading—health-care bills will soon rival mortgage bills in terms of dollar volume. As a result, look for more Americans to play Russian roulette with their health by opting out of the health-care system and not carrying insurance. This will lead to an epidemic of bankruptcies as non-insured Americans will be unable to cover the costs of heart surgery, cancer treatment, or other health-care procedures. According to the U.S. Surgeon General's Office, one in four (sixty million) non-elderly Americans will experience a gap in health coverage, and at least thirty million will be uninsured for one entire year. The result? Medical bills will become a leading cause of personal bankruptcy. The *New York Times* reports that a review of the last 300 bankruptcy cases in Arkansas showed a medical bill in half of them.

Retirees will be hardest hit by the rise in health-care costs. According to a recent study from Fidelity Investments, a couple retiring today at age sixty-five would need approximately $160,000 in savings to cover their retirement medical expenses, assuming that they do not have an employer-sponsored plan. With health-care costs rising anywhere from 7 to 15 percent per year (depending on which study you use), that figure will equal $500,000 to $2,225,000 respectively in twenty years.

So if you are forty-five years of age and looking to retire at age sixty-five, don't count on any retirement health insurance benefits. Corporate America will have long since passed that responsibility over to you. Financial planners in America currently create and administer retirement models that grossly misjudge the rising cost of treating chronic illness. Financial security, even avoiding bankruptcy as a senior, will for the first time include a vigilant focus on heath and wellness.

4. Health Care Will Be "Scored."

I once spoke with an elderly friend who indicated that in his time there was no such thing as a credit report. The idea of a national agency or agencies keeping track of how you paid your bills was just unheard of. Of course, he saw the creation and evolution of credit reports. After credit reports, we saw creditors concerned because they couldn't get enough rich data to find out more about people. How much money do they make? Where do they live? How much credit do they already have access to? Consequently, over the last several years a comprehensive credit score program has evolved.

Much like our current credit scoring system today, Americans will soon be "rated" by health-care insurers on the level of their health—good or bad. Factors comprising the score's formula will include medical history, genetic-risk factors, occupation, age, gender, race, body fat, and many other personal health-related factors. A high or "good health" score will send you to the front of the line for health-care insurance. A low score, however, may result in denied access to health-care coverage. Soon we'll see Americans fretting about their "health ratings" every bit as much as they do over their credit ratings and driving records. Not only will health insurers use health scores to gauge your health risk levels, but also employers and bankers will use them to calculate your long-term employability and financial stability.

In a deal that government will strike with the private sector for their ability to bear the newly acquired burden of health insurance for all workers, employers will be allowed to minimize their coverage risk through the implementation of this health score. As an example of how this prediction already shapes one area of insurance, look at the process of qualifying for life insurance. In predominantly all cases before any insurance is offered, a nurse practitioner will ask you a lot of very personal health questions, take all your vital signs, and draw blood for an in-depth clinical analysis. All of this data is then compiled into a risk analysis report that governs the financial level at which the insurance company will insure your life. We already have a "health score" model in life insurance and can expect to see richer data being used in the makeup of these health scores.

5. HVS Programs Will Share the Costs of Benefits.

In the future we will see insurance companies rewarding individuals through HVS—Health Value Score—pro-

7

grams. Through such programs, coverage premiums will be based on health scores, health insurance utilization, and other factors including wellness program participation and improvement from health base line. Patients will receive a refund or pay a penalty based on usage and health scores. American families will begin to look at their HVS ratings with the same interest and intensity they view their tax returns.

Sound far-fetched? We're already seeing the beginnings of such a program in many companies. With insurance rates climbing at double-digit rates annually, companies are becoming increasingly interested in the health of their employees. In an effort to lower costs and improve worker health, many employers—to the tune of 42 percent in America—are offering incentives and disincentives based on health behavior.

According to a recent article in *USA Today*, here are a few examples of what some companies are doing:

- American Cast Iron Pipe in Birmingham, AL, offers workers up to $200 in cash bonuses for not smoking and keeping their blood pressure, cholesterol, and weight within healthy limits.
- Employees at Logan Aluminum in Russellville, KY., receive $200 for filling out a health risk assessment and receive a shared year-end bonus if the company's overall health expenditures are controlled.
- Hannaford, a 119-store supermarket chain in the Northeast, offers a $15 a week discount on health insurance to non-smoking employees.
- Johnson and Johnson offers a $500 medical insurance discount to employees that participate in its wellness program.
- Pregnant women covered by health benefits at E.A.

Miller, a beef-packing plant in Hyrum, UT, are required to attend two prenatal classes and visit their doctor during the first trimester, or the company will not cover birth costs.

- Again at E.A. Miller, employees not wearing seatbelts when involved in auto accidents can expect to foot the bill for their injuries.

With Johnson and Johnson reporting an estimated savings of $8.5 million annually since the inception of its wellness program, it won't be long before more and more companies jump on the bandwagon. As Howard Leach, human resources manager for Logan Aluminum, puts it, "The secret of health care is not passing along costs to employees. The secret is asking employees to take control of their health."

Within a few years we will begin to see more and more of these incentive and disincentive programs develop—with even more wide-ranged effect. For example, a family that visits the doctor's office or utilizes the insurance's services only three times a year could qualify for a rebate for staying healthy. Their neighbors might be required to fork over a penalty for their abundant use of coverage. HVS will simply shift the burden of health care to those that utilize it most frequently and away from those who work to stay healthy.

6. More "Sicker and Quicker."

Most likely you haven't heard the term "sicker and quicker." Don't worry, you will. Sicker and quicker refers to the practice of health-care providers (especially hospitals) discharging patients that are not reimbursement favorable so they can make more money by reducing their level of care to "uninsured bodies." A RAND study found that in response to a change in the way

Medicare pays hospitals, patients are admitted "sicker" and released "quicker and sicker." In other words, future admittance policies will require a patient to be much sicker, while at the same time patients will be discharged when they meet criteria for what once constituted admittance into the hospital.

Let's take a look at how this might play out. On a sickness scale of one to ten, you show up at the hospital registering a "four." The admittance process determines you are not sick enough for hospital care. You return home where your condition unfortunately worsens to a "seven." Your second visit to the hospital results in admittance. Over the next twenty-four hours the doctors contain the condition back to the original level of "four" and then discharge you "sicker and quicker."

This does not mean that doctors are going to care less nor will they offer poor care. This is a reflection of cost-centered treatment. Older patients can also expect to bear the brunt of this cost-cutting trend as degenerative diseases such as arthritis, Alzheimer's, and macular degeneration fall from the list of disorders that "merit" treatment. You can also look for an increase in the denial of expensive treatments to so-called "non-productive" patients—patients who do not represent a source of reimbursement to the hospitals—in the next decade.

7. Health-Care Providers Will "Recycle" to Cut Costs.

Ever hear the term "reposable" before? Unfortunately, health-care providers will have to begin reusing disposable medical products in the coming years to help mitigate the rising price of health care. Other ways that health-care providers will cut costs will be to provide less time for patients with their care-givers and adapt a "cost-centered" versus "outcome-focused" financial framework for health care.

Many of my patented medical products are microsurgical scalpels. It is critical that scalpels used in microsurgery—especially surgery on the eye—be precisely sharp. Believe it or not, in America today, we are selling products to hospitals that are single-use disposables that are being used on as many as twenty patients per day. Does this practice save hundreds of dollars? No! Reusing disposables saves only a few dollars per patient—literally a couple of dollars.

The reason? Third-party providers that insure hospitals and day surgery centers pay what is called a global reimbursement fee. With these global reimbursement fees, the government is basically saying, "We are going to write you a check for $800 for that surgical case, and you can use that money to buy the necesary equipment and pharmaceuticals. What you use that money for doesn't matter to us. Do the surgery, but that is all we are paying—a flat global fee."

It's not uncommon to go into a surgery where they choose not to use certain types of medicines, which deepen the chamber during cataract surgery making the surgery easier and safer, because they are very expensive. Most ophthalmologists would agree that these drugs provide a better case, but they are used very sparingly and in many cases not at all in order to reduce costs. Additionally, they take single-use scalpels and autoclave them to be used again.

What's the risk? Without good sterile protocol, this process creates an unnecessary risk of cross-contamination for the patient. Another risk is having a blade that is dulled every time it is exposed to the high temperatures of the autoclave, which considerably reduces the functionality of the scalpel after each sequential use. We're not talking about what is happening in a third-world country—this is happening right here in America.

The past century has seen incredible advances in the treatment aspect of medicine. What has not been readily apparent is the comfortable rut that we have pounded out as we've walked the paths of health. As a society, we've come to believe, and even expect, that modern medicine will develop a miracle pill that will cure all our woes. Unfortunately, such is not the case. What we are beginning to see is that we have been circling the answer all along.

One of my favorite parables is the story of the processional caterpillars. Jean Henri Fabre spent hours experimenting with a line of processionary caterpillars. In one experiment, he coaxed the caterpillars onto the rim of a large flowerpot. He got the first caterpillar in line to follow the last and thus created a circle. Fabre's assumption that the caterpillars would soon figure out the trick and move to the flower in the middle of the pot was proven wrong. The habit of following the leader caused these caterpillars to follow each other around the rim of the pot for a full seven days. Starvation and exhaustion finally halted the march, but not before the damage was done.

For many years we've been following the circular pattern of treating symptoms as they appear. A symptom pops up, and we cover it with drugs and therapies designed to relieve the symptom. But what about the disease? Truly curbing the disease process—not simply easing the symptoms—can only occur when prevention is equally balanced with treatment.

That is the message of these predictions. Living on the safe side of these predictions will require that you step outside your current lifestyle habits and make the proper course corrections toward better health.

Chapter Two

We Super-Size Americans, Don't We?

"In the year 2000, the U.S. food industry provided 3,900 calories per person per day"

— BUSINESS WEEK

I have an identical twin. Having a twin grants you with a unique glimpse at your physiological photocopy. You experience firsthand what your life would be like if you had made different lifestyle choices, good or bad.

In high school, I chose to become a lifeguard and get involved with competitive swimming. Charlie, my twin, chose a musical path with his band that included too many late night pizzas. As a result of those early decisions, I became actively involved with fitness, whereas Charlie did not. For two decades, I watched the physical degradation of my own biological photocopy. By our twenties, Charlie weighed seventy-five pounds more than me and lived a very sedentary lifestyle. On the other hand, I became a vegetarian and continued an active lifestyle.

While visiting Charlie's family for Christmas, I sat down with him and asked, in essence, what his current lifestyle cost him. Charlie, a successful businessman, thought for a moment. Before I tell you what Charlie said, ask yourself the same question. What does your current lifestyle cost you? The answer may be a wake-up call—just as it was for my brother.

Charlie told me that he felt imprisoned by seventy-five pounds of cellulite. He felt it wasn't possible for him to feel good. As for the financial cost, the unpredictable expense of innumerable visits to the doctor's office and pharmacy during the upcoming years of inevitable high blood pressure, high cholesterol, and throbbing joint pain could easily surpass the cost of a new SUV.

After our conversation I went home and didn't see Charlie for a while. During this time, Charlie transformed himself from someone who mostly sat around to a pro-active, health-conscience individual. He reduced his portion size to a third of what it was before. He started using dietary supplements to nourish his body, while at the same time he reduced his intake of fats, sugars and carbohydrates. My chin dropped to the floor in amazement the next time I saw Charlie. Aside from not recognizing the Charlie I knew from our talk a year earlier, I found myself looking at a happier, more energetic photocopy of myself.

"Charlie," I asked, "how did you do it?"

"Future Charlie," he answered.

"Future Charlie?" I replied, and then my biological twin taught me an invaluable life lesson.

"Yeah," he replied. "After talking with you, I wrote a letter to 'Future Charlie'. I told him on a series of note cards that I was going to make an investment. I told 'Future Charlie' that I was going to get in shape by getting up everyday to work out. I promised him I would do whatever it took to nourish my body through supplements, a better diet, and reduced portion sizes to make sure I could achieve this physiological challenge. I committed to 'Future Charlie' that in one year I was going to be as healthy as my identical twin biological copy, Nick. And I signed the letter as 'Historical Charlie.'"

He stopped for a moment and then said, "I am Future Charlie."

My entrepreneurial side—that part of me that watches, learns, and then solves problems—latched onto the magic of "Future Charlie." America is overburdened with too many "Historical Charlies." The ideology of treatment, and the resulting heavy reliance on that treatment, will always struggle in resolving lifestyle-driven disease processes. Charlie closed his unfavorable health gap by taking responsibility for his lifestyle. By committing to get in shape, to eat better, and to supple-ment—in short, to practice a healthier lifestyle—Charlie closed the gap that he perceived between himself and what he viewed as his healthier biological photocopy.

Historical America is also seventy-five pounds overweight, lethargic, and not looking so good. The government and cor-porate America cannot bear the financial burden of solving chronic illness. Nor will they. Like it or not, that burden—the cost of being sick—will only be solved by closing the health gap on an individual basis. This burden of personal responsibility faces a stiff headwind that is predominantly influenced by the treatment mentality within our current health-care system.

FROM OUR FRIENDS ACROSS THE POND

On January 15, 2003, two members of parliament in London, England, introduced a bill for increased funding for London's fabled West End theatre district. The debate was intense—and it took a bizarre twist.

It seems that many of the buildings of the West End the-atre district, built in the Victorian age, had seats that couldn't accommodate the wide girths of the 21st century theatergoers. But it wasn't the locals that parliament members were trying to accommodate. It was the tourists—specifically American tourists with big wallets and bigger backsides that require "super-sized" seats.

"Thousands of people travel to London every year... pri-marily—sometimes solely—to visit the West End theatres," said

Chris Bryant, a Labour Party legislator from Wales in a February 2003 story on CNN.com entitled *Big Yanks Give U.K. Theatres Bum Rap.* "They see some wonderful shows, but because thirty-seven of London's theatres are either Victorian or Edwardian, they must see them in terrible buildings whose seats were built for backsides of the Victorian rather than the modern era—indeed, rather than for Americans."

So it's come to this. The land of milk and honey has turned into the land of cookie dough and hot buffalo wings. After years of lousy eating habits, Americans' backsides are catching up to them...literally. Foreign governments are actually looking to use scarce taxpayer funds to build wider seats to accommodate the extra layers of fat Americans have accumulated.

But it's not just our friends in the U.K. Back in the U.S., Southwest Airlines recently made headline news by politely— but firmly—suggesting that overweight travelers purchase not one but two seats for flight travel. The company wasn't being boorish about the request. It simply pointed out that it is "necessary" for "people of size" to buy the extra seat so as not to squeeze other passengers who might otherwise be sardined in next to them. Southwest even used politically correct code words in their press release announcing the new "full-figure fare" program. The program asks for the purchase of an additional seat "if the customer's girth is larger than one aircraft seat."

It's not just our image that's suffering from our super-sized diets. Obesity and that extra girth have been linked to a number of diseases, including cancer, cardiovascular disease and diabetes. If we're not careful, we'll find that not only will we need extra-large seats; we'll also need extra-large coffins.

THE CAUSE IS ALSO THE CURE

Diet is the key to preventing disease in our culture. Healthy eating, a solid regimen of exercise and dietary supplements are the key ingredients to good health. Unfortunately, to Americans that line of thought is hard to swallow—blaspheme in a fast food, microwave-maniacal land where nothing (as long as it's sweet and sugary) is too hard to swallow. After all, it's not polite, in this politically correct age, to point out that our population is gaining weight, that it needs to loosen a few notches on its collective belt and that a fresh look at our dietary habits may be in order.

That's a crime, especially when we consider the danger our children are in as a result of poor dietary habits. It's up to us— the adults—to curb this slide. But that's not the way many Americans see things. Mesmerized by Madison Avenue-fueled marketing campaigns where slim and hip actors extol the virtues of a supreme pizza or where thin, gorgeous models dance across our screen eating double cheeseburger, the ramifications of such a diet are overlooked—for our children and for ourselves. Nowhere in the ads does it tell viewers about the unhealthy fat content of such foods or of the dietary dangers that lurk as a result of eating them too often.

What goes unacknowledged by the fast-food industry as well as other promoters of unhealthy industries is the eventual price tag, both financially and physically, of indulging in such unhealthy lifestyles.

FAST FACTS: Super-Sized Nation
- Almost two-thirds of all Americans are overweight.
- Four percent of adolescents now have type II diabetes.
- Sugar is the number one food additive and is now included in foods such as bread, luncheon meat, canned vegetables, and mayonnaise.
- Americans are eating 500 more calories a day than they were back in 1984.

- One fast-food company's original meal of a 12-ounce soft drink, small fries and a hamburger provided 590 calories while their super-size "value" meal, complete with quarter-pound burger with cheese, super-size fries and drink, serves up 1,550 calories.
- Food companies spend $1.54 billion annually for advertisements promoting prepared, processed, and convenience foods.

Spake, Amanda. "A Fat Nation." U.S. News & World Report, August 19, 2002.

A DOUBLE-EDGED SWORD

According to an analysis by Anne Wolf of the University of Virginia, obesity costs around $118 billion annually. Adding obesity to the list of conditions covered by insurance would raise health insurance prices incredibly:

- If only 25 percent of the fifty-four million obese Americans visited the doctor only one time in the year and insurance covered it, the cost for insurance companies would be more than $810 million based on a charge of $60.
- A yearlong basic nutrition/behavior modification treatment program for those same people would run up the bill an estimated $450 per person.
- If just 10 percent of obese people went on prescription medication, the cost could be as much as $5.2 billion a year.
- Gastric bypass surgery for just 100,000 obese people would cost $2.4 billion.

That additional charge would result in higher premiums for everyone. But is that cost justifiable? Is the cost of treating obesity something that should be paid for regardless of the price tag?

"Everyone is concerned if they set a precedent, it's going to break the bank. My feeling is that obesity is going to break the bank if they don't do something," said James Hill, director of the Center for Human Nutrition at the University of Colorado Health Sciences Center. "Right behind this obesity epidemic is a diabetes epidemic, and that is very expensive."

Just how expensive will that diabetes epidemic be? The American Diabetic Association reported the following direct and indirect costs for 2002:

Direct Costs
- Direct medical expenditure for diabetes reached an estimated $91.8 billion in 2002 (compared to the $44 billion in 1997).
- Diabetes costs in 2002 represented 19 percent of personal health-care expenditures in the U.S., yet diabetics only account for 4.2 percent of the total U.S. population.
- Diabetes-related hospitalization totaled 16.9 million days, while physician visits to treat diabetes topped 62.6 million.

Indirect Costs
- Total indirect costs were estimated at $39.8 billion for 2002.
- Diabetes accounted for 88 million disability days.
- Permanent disability cases caused by diabetes rose to 176,000 at a cost of $7.5 billion.

The question then becomes: If we can't afford to pay for obesity treatment, can we afford to pay for the resultant diabetes treatment?

HIGH FAT, HIGH COSTS

How bad is it? Obesity contributes more to higher cost increases for health-care services and medications than do either smoking or problem drinking, according to a 2002 report published in the journal *Health Affairs*. The study compares the effects of obesity, smoking and problem drinking on health-care utilization and health status and concludes that obesity is associated with a 36 percent increase in in- and outpatient expenditures and a 77 percent increase in medication costs compared to people falling within a normal weight range.

Compare that to the long-term health-care problems associated with smoking and drinking. While it's no secret that both habits are debilitating and dangerous, problems associated with smoking and drinking aren't as severe as the problems associated with obesity. In the same *Health Affairs* study, smokers saw health-care price increases of only 21 percent for services and 28 percent for medications over those of non-smokers. Problem drinkers fared even better, so to speak.

{DEFINITION} According to the National Institutes of Health, anyone with a body mass index (a ratio between your height and weight) of twenty-five or above is considered overweight. Anyone with a body mass index of thirty or above is considered obese.

The result? The toll that obesity is taking on not only our populace but on our health-care system is mounting. "Obesity appears to have a stronger association with the occurrence of chronic medical conditions, reduced physical health-related quality of life, and increased health care and medication expenditures than smoking or problem drinking. Only twenty years' aging has similarly-sized effects," said study author Roland Sturm. According to Sturm, one in five Americans is obese, while an additional one in three is overweight. In addition, obesity has increased by 60 percent between 1991 and 2000, while smoking rates have been cut roughly in half since 1964.

The slippery slope America is on with its nutrition habits could have adverse effects on society for generations. According to a report by the Surgeon General's office, health problems resulting from being overweight and obese could reverse many of the health gains achieved in the U.S. in recent decades.

The report, entitled "The Surgeon General's Call to Action to Prevent and Decrease Overweight and Obesity," outlines strategies that communities can use in helping to address the problems. Those options include requiring physical education at all school grades, providing more healthy food options

"The Surgeon General's Call to Action to Prevent and Decrease Overweight and Obesity"

- In 1999, an estimated 13 percent of children and adolescents were overweight.
- Obesity among adults has doubled since 1980, while overweight among adolescents has tripled.
- Only 3 percent of all Americans meet at least four of the five federal Food Guide Pyramid recommendations for the intake of grains, fruits, vegetables, dairy products and meats.
- Less than one-third of Americans meet the federal recommendations to engage in at least 30 minutes of moderate physical activity at least five days a week, while 40 percent of adults engage in no leisure-time physical activity at all.
- Obesity trends are associated with dramatic increases in conditions such as asthma and type II diabetes in children.

on school campuses, and providing safe and accessible recreational facilities for residents of all ages.

"Overweight and obesity may soon cause as much preventable disease and death as cigarette smoking," Surgeon General David Satcher said. "People tend to think of overweight and obesity as strictly a personal matter, but there is much that communities can and should do to address these problems."

According to the report, approximately 300,000 U.S. deaths a year are associated with obesity and overweight (compared to more than 400,000 deaths a year associated with cigarette smoking). The total direct and indirect costs attributed to overweight and obesity amounted to a whopping $117 billion in the year 2000—enough to build 5,000 new schools, equip them with the latest computers and technology equipment and fully staff each one with fifty new teachers.

THE IMPACT ON OUR KIDS

The onset of obesity is a serious threat to our nation's children and our legacy. The effects of potato chips and soda for lunch multiple times a week are just starting to surface. We must act now before it's too late. Already we're seeing poor diets and sedentary lifestyles negatively impacting our children in the following ways:

- 80 percent of five to eight year olds have one risk factor for heart disease.
- 40 percent of five to eight year olds already exhibit obesity and high cholesterol levels.
- An obese preschooler has a 25 percent higher chance of being obese as an adult than does a non-obese child.
- 25 percent of second graders can't touch their toes.
- 76 percent of elementary school kids cannot do one chin-up.

- 50 percent of all teenage boys and 33 percent of teenage girls cannot walk up and down stairs for more than six minutes without straining their cardiovascular system.
- 30 percent of boys under thirteen cannot run a mile in less than ten minutes.

Unfortunately, unhealthy lifestyles, like inheritances and heirlooms, can be easily passed down from generation to generation. Many busy parents who value convenience think nothing of sending "Junior" off to fourth grade with a lunch box full of calorie-laden foodstuffs that fail to meet even minimum dietary guidelines.

When my daughter was in kindergarten, they would have a "share day" each week when each child had the opportunity to bring in their favorite treat. Inevitably, that treat was doughnuts, candy or cookies. Since our last name starts with a "W," it took a while before it was my daughter's turn. By the time her turn came around, I think that half of the kids in her class had developed type II diabetes.

When Taylor came in, she brought a case of navel oranges. We received a phone call that afternoon from her teacher. She said, "That was the most interesting phenomenon that has ever occurred in the 19 years that I have been teaching kindergarten. The kids had so much fun. There wasn't one kid in the class that didn't eat that treat."

Our children's bodies thrive on healthy foods. So where do they pick up these bad eating habits?

Consider, for example, the trendy "ready-to-go" lunches for children. They are one of the hottest-selling products in the food-services industry. To keep the money spigot flowing, the prepared-food industry has begun rolling out a super-sized version of their ready-to-go lunch packages for kids. Many of these super-sized products offer 40 percent more food than the original products with significantly higher calorie and fat contents as well. The prepared-food industry is hardly alone. Several fast-food giants have recently introduced "Big Kids" versions of their popular kid's meal menu options.

Moreover, what message do we send our children as they readily access vending machines for their school lunch with the $2.50 we give them when they leave home each morning? We send our children to school to learn, but what lesson is being taught when around virtually every corner they are greeted by a colorful and brightly lit vending machine crying out for their money? The idea started out with grand plans. The placement of soda and candy machines in schools provided an additional stream of badly needed revenue to pay for under-funded sporting, cheerleading and extracurricular programs.

While those programs have enjoyed more funding, we are faced with an unexpected side effect. Childhood obesity, according to the Surgeon General, has reached "epidemic proportions." Since 1980, the number of obese children has more than doubled—nearly 15 percent of all children in the U.S. are considered obese. That may not seem so scary—they're just kids, right? But obesity can lead to a number of childhood diseases including diabetes, high cholesterol levels, high blood pressure, and fatty liver disease. Additionally, obesity as a child has been shown in a number of studies to be a precursor to adult obesity—which has been linked to heart disease and several types of cancer.

And it's not just children's health that's being affected. Their quality of life is also undermined. In a study reported in *The Journal of the American Medical Association*, researchers found that obese children were almost as likely to have a lower quality of life as children undergoing cancer treatment. They just aren't able to participate in the activities that other, healthier children can.

The problem is the calorie-dense, nutrient-deficient foods they are eating. In one value meal, children have already consumed their recommended daily allowance of calories, while getting nowhere near the amount of nutrients they need. The predominantly sedentary lifestyle of children isn't helping either. Portable Game Boys and DVDs have replaced the days of playing kick-the-can, pick-up ball games, and hopscotch. The stark reality is that kids today are getting more calories, less nutrients, and fewer activities. The result is "big" kids—only it's the wrong kind of big.

O.K., I'm a realist. It's never going to be easy to force kids to eat their carrots and peas. That's why the prepared-food industry doesn't have a "Mega Peas and Carrots" ready-to-go product. But bulking up junk food portions isn't going to make it any easier either. Many parents may not realize it—and hence the reason for this book—but the building blocks for heart diseases can occur much earlier in life than conventional wisdom allows. Studies published in the June 2000 *Harvard Health Letter* and in the August 2000 *Arteriosclerosis, Thrombosis, and Vascular Biology Journal* indicate that atherosclerosis (hardening of the arteries) can begin as early as age nine. Heart disease isn't the only concern. In 1999, pediatricians began reporting an alarming rise in the number of cases of type II diabetes in children.

It's also no secret that lifestyle and nutritional habits in adolescence can lay the groundwork for one's adult years. Studies clearly show that excess weight in adolescence is a risk factor for adult obesity.

Obviously, the stakes are high. So high that society is doing a tremendous disservice to its children by promoting unhealthy nutritional choices as "fun" and "super-delicious." More and more, today's "Playstation Generation" of children is already leading sedentary lifestyles compared to earlier generations. Making it more difficult for them to get a good, balanced diet is only pouring more fuel on the fire.

"Snack Tax"

While I admit to no political station, I am a father of three young children. My children, just like yours, walk through the school halls. I realize that profits earned from vending-machine revenue help create otherwise unavailable extracurricular activities. I do not believe that the solution is the complete removal of vending machines from schools. However, is there a lesson to be learned in the way cigarettes have been taxed over the last few decades?

Increased cigarette prices have acted as a deterrent for many people and as a catalyst to stop smoking for others. Would doubling the price of sodas while also introducing healthier options at a lower cost decrease consumption of carbonated sugar water while maintaining the critical profit stream necessary to fund extracurricular activities?

Let's play this scenario out with a can of X-brand soda. Suppose your cost for each can is 35 cents. Selling the can through the vending machine at 60 cents gives you a profit of 25 cents per can. By raising the price to $1, the school could weather a drop of consumption by 50 percent and still come out ahead by 30 percent more revenue. Now add in healthy choices at the original price of 60 cents, and you can exceed original profit margins while giving kids a healthy alternative. The same principle could also work with candy, chips and pastries. Rather than offering popular snack foods, refrigerated fruits, yogurts and other healthy alternatives could be provided.

With another entrepreneurial spin, you might also find local private-sector companies willing to sponsor the healthy-alternative, less-profitable machines and further make more money in the process.

This may sound outlandish, but the idea of taxing nutritionally poor foods has been around for quite a while. Kelly Brownell, who originally championed the idea of a "Twinkie tax", recently teamed up with Michael Jacobson, executive director of the Center for Science in the Public Interest. Already garnering some media coverage—Brownell's idea was number seven on US News and World Report's "16 Silver Bullets: Smart Ideas to Fix the World" (1998)—this new pairing has received even more media exposure:

- Newsweek, June 25, 2000: "Protecting our kids may ultimately require such [tax] initiatives."
- Roll Call, June 1, 2000: "Fat police testing fast-food restaurants and applying a cholesterol tax wouldn't be impossible."
- Reuters News Service, June 3, 2000: "A tax on snacks and soft drinks could be just the ticket to keep Americans slim and trim."
- The Associated Press, June 10, 2000: "Like fat creeping up on a person's thighs, a penny tax on junk food and soda would be little-noticed at first but have long-term impact."
- The Tampa Tribune, June 16, 2000: Business writer Mike Stobbe proposed a "very, very steep tax" on snack foods to "subsidize the costs of healthy foods." In fact, Stobbe called for such a high tax that you could possibly see "a $3.00 Snickers® bar."

WOULD YOU LIKE TO SUPER-SIZE THAT SERVING OF STRESS?

Eating too much and eating the wrong kinds of foods aren't the only bad habits many of us have picked up over the years. Our habit to let stress run and ruin our lives is also high on the list of modern killers.

While information technology has been a blessing to most, it is impacting American working professionals in ways we never imagined. Sure, information technology made us better workplace "producers," but that has meant bringing the workplace with us wherever we go, via laptop computers, personal digital assistants, cell phones, and fax machines.

Such high tech instruments were supposed to free us from the surly bonds of inefficiency. But in a pact that would make Machiavelli proud, we've traded higher productivity for a good chunk of our personal freedom. Think about it. Did you check e-mail on your last vacation? Do you bring your cell phone to dinner? Ball games? Your daughter's ballet recital?

Earlier generations weren't stressed like we are today. Twenty-five years ago the notion of being wired into your workplace from your home, your car, or from 30,000 feet above Detroit was a fantasy. Your dad may have brought home a briefcase crammed with paperwork once in a while, but it was the exception rather than the rule. The advent of technology, which among other delights promised to abolish the paper-strewn office and replace it with a digital one we could carry with us, has seemingly placed all of us on a 24/7 on-call basis.

Couple the work stress that we all feel with the specter of terror we've lived under since September 11th, and the continuing prospects of an uncertain geopolitical future, and you have the makings of a societal stress of epic proportions. And it shows. A study conducted by the manufacturers of Tylenol® indicates that a large number of Americans are experiencing mounting levels of stress and tension in their lives. The study—

called "The Tension Tracker 2002"—revealed that the top triggers of stress in America are lack of time because of excessive work, concern about terrorism, and finances.

Stress Inducers: Data from the Tension Tracker 2002

Americans are apparently an increasingly anxious lot. Here are the top reasons why, according to Tylenol's Tension Tracker 2002 Study:

Time—Lack of time was named by 62 percent of those surveyed as a great source of stress; many Americans say it's because they have too much work or work too many hours. In fact, U.S. workers put in more hours on the job than the labor force of any other industrial nation.

Terror—The events of September 11 loomed large to respondents. Over half of the survey participants (61 percent) named 9/11 and threats of terrorism as a great source of stress. Among them, 79 percent said the attacks of September 11 have changed America's way of life.

Tension—Among the 58 percent of Americans who name financial and money concerns as a source of tension, a majority listed not being able to save money, the high cost of living, not being able to pay bills on time and not being able to afford things they want as their main sources of stress. This is against a backdrop where personal savings as a percentage of disposable income has fallen sharply since the 1990, and the delinquency rate on credit cards is the highest since 1980.

It's not that stress is necessarily bad in and of itself. Stress can be good for your physical and mental health. The problems start when stress becomes an unrelenting monster that is constantly breathing down your neck.

Let's look at an example from Shawn Talbott, Ph.D. If you were to go to Africa, you would no doubt see zebras sometime during your trip. If you were lucky, you might also witness a lion hunting that zebra. When the lion strikes, the zebra will go through a natural response that you learned about in school— fight or flight. Recognizing the threat of the lion, the zebra's brain will release a message that starts a neurological, biochemical, hormonal, and physiological response to the threat. This response will give the zebra that little burst of energy that we associate with stressful situations—the muscles will get revved and running, the heart will pound, and senses will become more acute. All of this is designed to make a get-away from the lion.

The difference between the zebra's stress and our "human" stress is that the zebra's ends. Once the zebra has gotten away— if he's lucky—his body will relax, hormone levels will drop, and the zebra will go back to normal.

Contrast that with our modern lifestyles. Sure, we have the occasional momentary stressor—like when a car swerves in front of you or you drop a china dish. But we also have other, more long-lasting stressors— like the mortgage, the car payment, your job, credit card payments, and any other number of long-term stresses. These stressors stay with us all day, everyday. With these constant stressors, your body's stress response is always on alert so you never relax. Your heart rate stays sky-high, your hormones stay at elevated levels, and your brain is constantly firing trying to find a way to end the stress. It's very similar to putting the emergency brake on in your car, and then slipping it into gear and flooring the gas pedal without ever releasing the brake. Your car is working extra hard but not getting anywhere. Sooner or later, something will give.

Relieving stress from your life becomes vitally important when you consider just how much damage chronic or long-term stress can do. Many of us suffer from illnesses that could be relieved by simply alleviating the stress we suffer from. Surveys show between 60 and 90 percent of visits to primary care physicians are for stress-related problems.

The Cortisol Connection

Shawn Talbott, PhD, has written an excellent book on stress and how it not only makes you fat but also ruins your health. According to the research that Talbott explores in his book, when you are under stress, your body releases a hormone called cortisol. Cortisol regulates your body's metabolism of glucose, protein and fatty acids. It also has important functions in mood control, inflammation, immune cells, blood and blood vessels, and the maintenance of connective tissues like bone, muscles and skin. Cortisol also plays a role in the "fight-or-flight" response.

But when we are regularly and repeatedly exposed to this stress hormone, we will begin to deteriorate. When faced with stress, cortisol loads your blood with fat and glucose in order to facilitate the fight-or-flight response. Imagine what happens when you have cortisol filling your blood with fat and sugar all day long. The effects on your organs and body are horrendous! In short, cortisol is slowly wearing us down and making us fat at the same time.

SEDENTARY LIFESTYLES

While poor nutrition and increased stress are proving to be the cornerstones of increasingly unhealthy lifestyles for Americans, one solution that's readily available—exercise—is being mostly overlooked.

Longer hours in the workplace, the exhaustion of coming home and caring for the children, and a culture that makes it ever so easy to flop down on the couch in our free hours and click our way through 225 channels of satellite television have all combined to chip away at our once robust and healthy resolve to keep fit and look good.

A sedentary lifestyle only ups the ante in terms of contracting chronic diseases. Medical experts have long noted that physical activity has been found to promote good health and build a muscular barrier against obesity and its close culture of chronic diseases including heart disease, diabetes, hypertension, and cancer.

Still, we're either too tired or too unwilling to strap on the jogging shoes or jump in the pool for a few laps. Our sedentary lifestyles, combined with other unhealthy lifestyles, are increasing the speed in which Americans are sliding into a new existence of sickness.

FAST FACTS: The High Cost of Being Unhealthy

Our unhealthy lifestyles are taking a toll on our health-care system. Consider these figures from the U.S. Surgeon General's Office:

- Adults' poor nutrition habits are linked to $146 billion in medical costs per year (almost 15 percent of an estimated total national medical expenditure of $1 trillion).
- American adults' sedentary lifestyle adds upward of $76.6 billion in yearly direct-medical costs (2000).
- In the U.S., health-related costs due to overweight and obesity are estimated at $117 billion (2000).

- The cost of chronic disease in the U.S. is more than half a trillion dollars.

SUMMARY

Poor eating habits, high levels of stress and the lack of exercise all contribute to the lousy nutritional and lifestyle habits many Americans now have. All of these issues also point to high costs financially, physically and emotionally for millions of Americans. Take a moment to think about the following facts:

- According to an article in the January/February issue of *Health Affairs*, U.S. health-care spending increased from $1.3 trillion in 2000 to $1.4 trillion in 2001—a health-care cost of about $5,035 per person on an annual basis.
- A huge chunk of the U.S. state-by-state budget deficit issues can be placed on the doorstep of high health-care costs. Overall, health care represents about 30 percent of the average state budget. Medicaid alone accounts for 20 percent of that outlay. Total health-care costs are growing at about four times the rate of inflation.

Chapter Three

Remodel Your Life

For sixteen years, researchers at Harvard Medical School and the Dana Farber Cancer Institute in Boston, MA, evaluated 900,000 people who, at the study's conception, were cancer free. At the end of the study, the researchers concluded that excess weight might account for more than 90,000 cases of cancer each year. According to the study, losing weight could prevent one of every six cancer deaths in the U.S. "What's clear is that large studies of this sort—and this is the biggest and best to date—show very clearly [obesity] is a major health problem in this country," said Dr. Robert Mayer of Harvard Medical School and the Dana Farber Cancer Institute.

One in six cancer deaths could be prevented by losing weight. That's an incredible statistic. But that's not all. Increased waistlines also increase our risks of other diseases, like cardiovascular disease and diabetes. Something has to change. The good news is that it's not too late...yet.

Perhaps the greatest contributor to our situation today is ignorance. Our society has become numb to the barrage of daily newsbreaks, national studies, and infomercials. While closing our ears to the hyperbole and hype, we miss the basics, the solutions, and the simple message that prevention stands as our most formidable ally.

Perhaps our most difficult challenge is breaking our current lifestyle habits. Waking up late, quick and easy sugar-based cereals, carbonated sugar water and fries, taking the elevator instead of the stairs and choosing to watch primetime instead of living it—each contains an opportunity for change, to take a step in a better direction. This book is not about a destination. Rather, it is about living a more purposeful journey.

Birthdays will come; anniversaries will pass. The question you must ask is how you will look at those moments. Start building into your mind ways that you and your family can take steps toward the magic of your own "Future Charlie." As I related in chapter two, my twin brother, Charlie, decided that he wouldn't procrastinate his journey to better health any longer. In a year's time he made incredible progress down that road. And here's the good news—so can you.

When you think about it, there's no magic elixir involved. To feel better we have to start living better. Ask any doctor. "It's no secret," said Mark Stafford, M.D., associate professor of internal medicine at University of Alabama at Birmingham and author of *Maximal Living*, a weekly online health column. "Based on 20 years of caring for patients, I've observed that people who achieve and enjoy life the most share 10 simple habits: eat a balanced diet; exercise regularly; maintain a healthy body weight; sleep at least seven hours a night; do things in moderation avoiding extremes; don't take life too seriously; have at least one close, personal friend; have a healthy, loving relationship with a higher power; resolve conflicts quickly; and live in the moment, celebrating life." There's always room for improvement and I would add an additional item to the list.

As a vegetarian and avid outdoor enthusiast, I had always discounted the need for supplementation. I inaccurately thought that a good diet alone contained the nutrients my body needed to provide protection against the conditions our nation suffers from.

Springtime in Northern California has always meant allergies for me. Not a week into my new supplement regimen, I, for the first time, was awakened by the smell of my automatic coffee maker. I can't provide you any science for this phenomenon. All I know is the most popular allergy medications on the market never provided me a morning free from congestion.

I find this experience remarkable. I had been living a life that by all standards was healthier than most. Yet by adding a simple practice that I had never believed necessary, my body was able to solve its own problem without the aid of pharmaceutical treatment. And best of all, I created a new, constructive habit that didn't require a complete remodeling of my lifestyle.

Here's the rub. Supplementation can benefit anyone. Whether you have perfect eating habits, or you subsist off of cheeseburgers and fries, adding a quality supplement can immediately provide you with better health and added protection.

SUPPLEMENTATION

In a recent conversation with a leading expert in the field of nutrition, the benefits of supplementation were driven home even more. As we discussed nutrition the point was brought out that the average intake of fruits and vegetables is 2.3 servings a day. Yet the National Cancer Institute and the FDA's Food Guide Pyramid call for five to ten servings per day. What is even more shocking is that of those 2.3 servings of fruits and vegetables, the most popular fruit is the banana and the most popular vegetable is the potato in the form of a french fry! Neither of these foods has very high levels of nutrients. Plain and simple, we need to eat more fruits, vegetables, and whole grains.

But even if you are eating those servings of fruits and vegetables, you may still be lacking. "Let's say you're one of the 10 percent of Americans who does eat three to five vegetables daily. Do you still need a supplement?" asked Jeffrey Blumberg, PhD, an antioxidant researcher at Tufts University in Boston, MA. "Almost certainly because, on any given day, your choice among those foods is likely to fall short in something."

Better eating habits won't completely fill the void created by poor nutrition. That same conversation yielded the following reason why supplementation is absolutely critical. We can look at vitamin E for example. There is very good scientific and medical data that shows that 200 to 400 and even up to 800 international units (IU) of vitamin E can help prevent some cardiovascular complications. The Recommended Dietary Allowance for vitamin E is only 30 IUs. That's enough to prevent a deficiency, but it's certainly not the 300 IUs needed to protect against cardiovascular disease. You can eat a handful of nuts and fulfill the RDA for vitamin E. But to reach that protective level of 300 units, you would have to eat a whole bucket of almonds. That would also complicate weight-loss programs with an additional 10,000 calories.

We live in a world that uses the RDA as an acceptable nutritional benchmark. We have been indoctrinated to believe that if we meet those RDAs, we'll have good health. The actual story is much different. The RDAs were developed only to prevent deficiency disorders like scurvy, beriberi and rickets. We've already looked at the example of vitamin E. Protection against diseases from vitamin E starts at 300 IUs, yet the RDA is only 30 IUs—ten times less than what is needed. Vitamin E is but one case in an entire family of required nutrients.

Of course, that's assuming that foods actually have nutrients in them. Our farm soils are becoming increasingly low in nutrients. For instance, according to Harold D. Foster, PhD, a medical geographer and professor at the University of Victoria, Canada, soil in parts of the Northeast, Northwest, and Florida contain virtually no selenium. As a result, foods coming from those areas have no selenium either. Low-selenium diets increase your risk of cancer and in men increase chances of infertility. In addition, levels of water-soluble nutrients, especially vitamin C and the B vitamins, drop after harvesting and during storage, cooking, refrigeration, and reheating. According to Hugh D. Riordan, MD, head of the nonprofit Bright Spot for Health Clinic in Wichita, KA, cooking destroys half of the folic acid in food. Low levels of vitamin C and B—as well as folic acid—are indicative of increased risk of cardiovascular disease.

A recent article in *The Journal of the American Medical Association* further promotes supplementation. This article reported that the average American diet is sufficient to prevent deficiency disorders, but this same diet was resulting in "suboptimal levels of vitamins." The article went on to explain that "recent evidence has shown that suboptimal levels of vitamins, even well above those causing deficiency syndromes, are risk factors for chronic disease such as cardiovascular disease, cancer, and osteoporosis. A large proportion of the general population is apparently at increased risk for this reason…. *The high prevalence of suboptimal vitamin levels implies that the usual U.S. diet provides an insufficient amount of these vitamins*" (italics added). The article concludes by recommending that every adult should take a multi-vitamin daily.

ALWAYS EAT YOUR VEGGIES

Yet, supplementation alone is not the answer. We cannot simply add a quality supplement and expect it to counteract all the ill effects of a poor diet. The same article from *The Journal of the American Medical Association* stated, "Foods contain thousands of compounds that may be biologically active, including hundreds of natural antioxidants, carotenoids, and flavonoids.

For these reasons, vitamin supplementation is not an adequate substitute for a good diet."

Good eating habits are the cornerstone of improved health. You have to eat better if you want to live better. Our current habits are the product of years of "intake." Gradual change over time in the form of "baby steps" will remodel your lifestyle. As parents, this can start by cutting out the sugar cereals for breakfast, including actual fruit in lunches rather than "fruit snacks" and a policy that every evening meal includes at least one serving of vegetables, preferably fresh.

Unfortunately, as a nation we're not moving in that direction. Kim Feil, division president at Information Resources, which recently released a survey on the eating habits of 2000 consumers, said, "The fundamental definition of a meal has changed. Today, a meal can be a Diet Coke® and a Snickers® bar." The study found that 35 percent of Americans eat two or fewer "square" meals a day, while only 42 percent feel they have a well-balanced diet. Another study completed by Frito-Lay estimated that Americans skipped forty billion meals in 2002.

And here's the kicker: We may be skipping meals, but we're not eating less. In fact, we're consuming more calories than ever before. Rather than balanced meals, we've moved to a practice of "grazing." We grab snacks and quick meals here and there. But these "meals," while filling, are far from nutritious. Take, for instance, Cinnabon®. Cinnabon has 286 mall locations, eighty-four airport shops and another 100 sites in the works— all in places notorious for quick snacks. But eating just one Cinnabon cinnamon roll will provide you with 730 calories! That's one-third of the daily-recommended load of calories. But what if you wanted a Caramel Pecanbon™? Well, you just ate half of your calories—1100!

But that was just a snack, right? You'll still eat three meals a day in addition to grazing. "I don't call it grazing," said Marion Nestle, head of the nutrition department at New York University. "I call it eating too often and too much."

Yet for all our eating, we're still a nation that has "suboptimal levels" of vitamins in our systems. Fixing the problem, however, won't require a complete overhaul of your eating habits. The change to a better diet may be easier than you think.

A Dutch study that appeared in a recent issue of *The Journal of Nutrition* concludes that a diet that features five servings of fruits and vegetables daily can lead to a longer, healthier life. In the study, scientists selected forty-seven people who normally consumed a diet low in fruits and vegetables. They then assigned participants to consume either a standard Dutch diet that included a "low" amount (100 grams, or about one serving) of fruits and vegetables or a "high" amount (500 grams, or about five servings) of fruits and vegetables plus 200 ml (about 6.5 oz) of fruit juice. At the end of the four-week study, those in the "high" fruit and vegetable group had appreciably higher blood levels of several antioxidant nutrients, including beta-carotene, lutein, and vitamin C as well as moderate increases in folate—in short the stuff that disease prevention is made of.

A diet loaded with apples, oranges, bananas, and assorted other fruits can be beneficial to your body, particularly your heart. Researchers at the University of California, Davis School of Medicine found in a recent study that drinking apple juice and eating apples has a beneficial effect on risk factors for heart disease. The study shows that compounds in apples and apple juice act in much the same way that red wine and tea do to slow one of the processes that lead to heart disease. These compounds act as antioxidants to delay the breakdown of LDL or "bad" cholesterol. When LDL oxidizes, or deteriorates in the blood, plaque accumulates along the walls of the coronary artery and causes atherosclerosis.

More and more evidence is mounting in support of diets that feature fruits and vegetables. Although you may have been taught that the best diet is the USDA's Food Guide Pyramid, there is a rising movement stating that this diet is flawed. Most experts are now offering new guidelines—guidelines that focus on increased portions of fruits and vegetables.

Dr. Walter Willet and his colleagues at the Harvard School of Public Health are one group of experts who have developed a new eating guide. "The Healthy Eating Pyramid" came about after Dr. Willet and friends reviewed the data from the Nurses' Health Study, the Physicians' Health Study, and the Health Professional's Follow-Up Study. This new pyramid calls for increased consumption of whole-grain foods, plant oils and vegetables. According to the study, not only were adherents to Dr. Willet's pyramid healthier, they also lowered their risks of chronic disease (women following the plan suffer 28 percent

The Skin You're In

Save face by eating healthy. According to the Mayo Clinic Women's *HealthSource Special Report,* a diet rich in fruits and vegetables can improve the condition, tone and texture of your skin. In *The Journal of American College of Nutrition,* the same clinic cites a recent study of more than 400 people age 70 or older living in Australia, Sweden or Greece. The study found that whether they were fair skinned or dark skinned, people who ate a diet rich in green leafy vegetables, beans, olive oil, nuts and multi-grain breads, but skipped the butter, red meat and sugary goodies, were less susceptible to wrinkling. Researchers speculate that antioxidant vitamins, such as A, C and E, which are plentiful in protective foods, may help save your skin from environmental damage.

less heart disease—double the number of that of USDA guide-line followers). The American Institute for Cancer Research has also issued a new food guide that calls for vegetables, fruits, whole grains, and beans to cover two-thirds of your plate while animal source foods should cover only one-third.

Simply put, make a few minor changes in your diet, and you'll start feeling better, living longer, and looking healthier. Instead of reaching for that cola, grab a fruit drink. Replacing white bread with whole-grain breads will give you 200 to 700 percent more calcium, magnesium, phosphorous, potassium, zinc, copper, manganese, selenium, pantothenic acid, and vita-mins B6 and E.

Melding fruits and vegetables into your lifestyle isn't as dif-ficult as you might think. You just have to think creatively. Try these tips on for size:

- Bring some fresh or dried fruit with you to work, school, or wherever you have to go during the day.
- Out to eat? Hit the salad bar first. You may enjoy your meal so much that you'll never get to the cheeseburger or steak.
- Top off your breakfast cereal with a slice of fruit. A slice of banana, some fresh strawberries, or even some grapes make your cereal healthier and tastier.
- Combine the best of both worlds and make a salad out of fruits and vegetables. Throw some sliced oranges on that spinach salad and spice things up a bit. Or add raisins to your garden salad. Open up your mind and try some combinations of your own.
- Keep a bowl of fresh fruits and vegetables out on your kitchen counter at all times. That way when you're tempted to snack, some healthy foods are within easy reach.

Your Best Bets

According to the U.S. Food and Drug Administration, some fruits and some vegetables are better than others. Here is their list of the most effective foods from the fruits and vegetable families:

Fruits
Oranges
Strawberries
Kiwi
Cantaloupe
Peaches and nectarines
Grapes

Vegetables
Broccoli
Spinach
Red peppers
Sweet potatoes
Onions
Tomatoes

Fruits and vegetables are a critical component of your diet. But they're not everything. When it comes to a good, balanced diet, you have to develop the mindset that what you're eating has an impact, negative or positive, on your health.

HAVE DIET QUESTIONS? GET HELP

When it comes to planning their vacations, their careers, even their taxes, Americans have no problem seeking out a qualified professional to help them meet their goals. Why should something as important as our diet be any different? That's why I'm a big advocate of getting professional nutritional help to improve our eating habits. And I'm not alone.

According to a study by Massachusetts General Hospital, people who received dietary counseling to help them lower their cholesterol levels reported higher levels of satisfaction with their quality of life and health care than individuals who tried to lower their cholesterol in other ways. "Contrary to popular belief, there is no apparent reduction but rather an improvement in some measures of quality of life and patient satisfaction with medical nutritional therapy for high cholesterol," said Linda M. Delahanty, M.S., R.D., of the Diabetes Center of Massachusetts General Hospital.

Patients who received the medical nutritional therapy reported being more satisfied with their ability to manage their cholesterol, their health-care visits, their appearance and eating habits, and their overall health. The counseled group also said that they didn't feel deprived of their enjoyment of food, inconvenienced while shopping or preparing food, or restricted from eating out on their new diet plan.

And that's the whole point—changing your diet doesn't have to be an inconvenience. Nor does it need to be a matter of depriving yourself of those things you enjoy. Simple, minor changes and an overall awareness of better health is all it takes. You can do it!

GET THAT HEART PUMPING!

Of the three—supplementation, diet, and exercise—a meaningful exercise habit requires the greatest sacrifice. Waking up an extra 45 minutes early or trying to squeeze in a workout session before heading to bed is no small task. Exercise actively compensates the sacrifice with increased energy, improved self-confidence,

Guidelines for Eating Out

In a November 2002 study, Wake Forest University Baptist Medical Center nutritionist Mara Vitolins, Ph.D., said that it is possible to learn strategies to eat a healthy meal—even at a fast-food restaurant. Vitolins cited unique challenges including "biggie" portions, appetizers such as "blooming onions," desserts called "chocolate decadence," and pressure from friends to abandon good nutritional practices when dining out with the gang. Here are some tips from Vitolins when dining out:

1. **Call ahead.** "When going out to dinner at a restaurant, call the restaurant in advance to find out what types of healthier foods they have on the menu. This eliminates having to ask the wait staff about these items in front of your friends."

2. **Learn the lingo.** "Knowing that terms such as 'steamed,' 'poached,' or 'roasted'' indicate lower fat preparation methods whereas 'buttered,' 'escalloped,' 'au gratin,' or 'fried' indicate greater amounts of fat were used in the preparation can really make a difference in the amount of calories you consume. Asking for a baked potato to replace the escalloped potatoes can save you many calories, in particular, fat calories."

3. **Don't be afraid to ask.** Don't be afraid to modify. "Restaurant wait staff can assist you, but you have to ask. They can tell you about the types of sauces served on main dishes and lower calorie/fat dressing choices as well as options for side dishes. Feel free to modify your meal by asking for the sauce to be left off or served on the side, selecting a lower-fat dressing and/or asking for it on the side, leaving the grated cheese off your salad, and/or ordering sherbet without the cake. Most restaurants will accommodate these types of menu modifications, and if they don't, consider selecting a different restaurant the next time you go out to dine."

4. **Control your portions.** "At all costs, refrain from super sizing your order, even if there is economic incentive to do so. Order a kid's meal for the smaller portions, fewer calories, and less fat."

5. **Know your fast food restaurants.** "Some fast food restaurants have healthier food selections, such as baked potatoes (plain), chili, salads, or vegetarian burgers."

and better health. While setting a goal to run the local marathon in six months is admirable, look to slowly work into your life a habit of functional exercise.

Repeated studies are showing just how beneficial regular exercise is. In 1996, the Surgeon General released a report on physical activity and health. This report—coincidentally appearing the same year as the 100-year celebration of the Olympics and the 50-year anniversary for the Centers for Disease Control and Prevention—touted the health benefits of regular physical exercise. The report also displayed just how sedentary our nation has become. According to the report, more than 60 percent of Americans are not regularly active, while 25 percent of the adult population is not active at all.

And it's no wonder why. More and more, we live in an increasingly technologically advanced society. Anymore, physical activity is something that is completely unnecessary. We have motorized transportation to get us to and from any destination—even to get us up and down stairs. Sedentary activities are prolific, and very tempting. More and more people spend time watching television, surfing the net, playing video games, or simply not moving at all. We seem perfectly content to live our lives vicariously through others depicted on prime-time television in "real-life" shows while we let our own prime time escape us.

Unfortunately, all these wasted hours of physical inactivity are beginning to show. But it is a problem that can be corrected. By simply increasing how active you are you can begin to enjoy the same benefits as active people.

And what are those benefits? According to the American Council on Exercise, individuals who exercise regularly are less likely to develop:

- Heart disease
- Diabetes
- High blood pressure

- High cholesterol levels
- Certain forms of cancer
- Osteoporosis

And, people who exercise regularly are more likely to:

- Maintain a healthy weight
- Effectively control the pain and joint swelling that accompanies arthritis
- Maintain lean muscle—which is often lost with aging
- Have higher levels of self-esteem and self-confidence
- Continue to be active as they grow older
- Experience overall feelings of well-being and good health

Physical activity, according to the Surgeon General's report, has positive impacts on the musculoskeletal, cardiovascular, respiratory, and endocrine systems. Regular activity also reduces depression, anxiety, and stress while improving mood and enhancing a person's ability to perform daily tasks.

Chances are you've already witnessed firsthand these benefits. Whether it is you that is active or someone you know, you have seen the positive effects of activity. Active people radiate good health. They are sick less often; able to participate more, contribute more, and, in short, do more; for the most part they seem more successful; they have better relationships; they look and feel better; and the list could go on and on.

In my travels I have had the opportunity to stay in a number of hotels. When opportunity allowed, I've stayed in some of the nicest hotels available. I've also stayed in quite a few of the more economical models. I've witnessed an interesting phenomenon at these places. Inevitably, the nicer hotels, there is a line of people waiting to get into the workout facilities. On the other hand, at the lower-priced hotels, you could fire a cannon

Major Conclusions of The Surgeon General's Report on Physical Activity and Health:

1. People of all ages, both male and female, benefit from regular physical activity.

2. Significant health benefits can be obtained by including a moderate amount of physical activity—for example, thirty minutes of brisk walking or raking leaves, fifteen minutes of running, or forty-five minutes of playing volleyball—on most, if not all, days of the week. Through a modest increase in daily activity, most Americans can improve their health and quality of life.

3. Additional health benefits can be gained through greater amounts of activity. People who can maintain a regular regimen of activity that is of longer duration or of more vigorous intensity are likely to derive greater benefit.

4. Physical activity reduces the risk of premature mortality in general, coronary heart disease, hypertension, colon cancer, and diabetes mellitus in general. Physical activity also improves mental health and is important for the health of muscles, bones, and joints.

5. More than 60 % of American adults are not regularly physically active. In fact, 25 % of all adults are not active at all.

6. Nearly half of American youths 12-21 years of age are not vigorously active on a regular basis. Moreover, physical activity declines dramatically during adolescence.

7. Daily enrollment in physical education classes has declined among high school students from 42 percent in 1991 to 25 percent in 1995.

in any direction in the workout room and not hit a soul—yet these hotels have a plethora of satellite dishes on the roof ensuring that every room has hundreds of channels to choose from. While no direct correlation can be drawn between physical fitness and success, it seems to be that the vast majority of "successful" people are also physically successful.

This point cannot be stressed enough—exercise is vitally important. In fact, one entire chapter in the Surgeon General's report deals solely on exercise and the prevention of disease. Mentioned also in that chapter is the fact that exercise increases the quality of life. If you exercise, you'll see a dramatic improvement not only in your health, but also in how you feel and ultimately, how you live.

The current recommendation for activity is thirty minutes everyday. However, a recent report featured in *The Journal of the American Medical Association* reported that high-intensity exercise might be even more beneficial. Researchers found that men who exercised at high intensity were 17 percent less likely to develop heart disease than those who did low-intensity exercise.

Additionally, the study reported on the benefits of weight lifting. Researchers discovered that men who engaged in weight training for thirty minutes or more weekly had a 23 percent lower risk of heart disease than men who did not lift weights. The researchers theorized that the benefits of weight training might result from reductions in blood pressure and body fat brought about by weight training. Weight training has many other benefits as well. Load-bearing exercises have long been touted as a preventive measure for osteoporosis and arthritis. Weight training also increases and helps maintain range of motion—in fact one study found that Olympic weight lifters were second in flexibility only to gymnasts. Inflexibility and lowered motility are major factors in disability in the elderly. Finally, weight lifting increases the amount of lean muscle mass in the body. This translates into increased strength and a higher metabolism.

But don't let the thought that you have to be Herculean in your workouts to get any benefits scare you away from working out. Any activity is better than none. While high intensity runners are 42 percent less likely to develop heart disease compared to those who are not active, brisk walkers also enjoy the lowered probability of heart disease—they are 18 percent less likely to develop heart disease when compared to their sedentary counterparts.

If you're still scared of getting up and sweating out the miles, there's good news for you yet. The recommendation of thirty minutes of daily activity is a cumulative measurement, not a one-shot deal. You can add up short, ten minute bouts of exercise to reach your daily goal. So instead of pounding out the miles a half hour at a time, you can take quick ten minute walks or short bursts of weight lifting several times throughout the day and still reap the same benefits as the health nuts in the gym. Granted, the gym enthusiasts will enjoy a higher level of those benefits, but every little bit counts. And even more motivating is that you need not feel that you have to be out there running or lifting weights. Common activities can be beneficial as well. Gardening, mowing the lawn, shoveling snow off the driveway, and housecleaning can qualify as physical activity. Any activity that gets your heart pumping will provide you some benefit. The key is to make sure you get at least thirty minutes of activity everyday. You may end up with the most beautiful lawn on the block or the cleanest house in the neighborhood, but chances are you won't complain about those fringe benefits.

On a less positive note, the legacy that we are passing on to our children has led to an epidemic of adolescent obesity and weakness. A fitness-testing program run by the Chrysler Fund Amateur Athletic Union, which tracks the fitness levels of 9.7

million American youths between the ages of six and seventeen, shows that children are getting slower and weaker. Since 1980, there has been a 10 percent drop in distance run scores and an 11 percent decline in the number of children who scored "satisfactory" on the entire test. Something has got to change.

Rather than allowing life to simply pass us by, we should get out and start living our lives. I'm willing to bet that your memories are stocked full of experiences with family and friends as you camped, played sports, went on picnics and hikes, and just had fun. What memories are our children building? When they are parents will they look back and remember the time that you took them swimming in the lake, or will they be able to recite every password to every video game from their era? Will they remember the time they hit the winning homerun, or will they be able to describe in detail Kramer's antics on Seinfeld? The joy of physical activity is not necessarily the health benefits that accompany such activities, but rather the memories that will stay with you long after the game has ended.

IT'S UP TO YOU

While touching on three vital areas to increased health—supplementation, diet, and exercise, I haven't offered a cookie-cutter program. Instead of trying to develop some plan that will map out your every step on the journey, I've tried to supply you with a valuable assortment of facts. You can set your own course. You know your needs better than anyone else, and so only you are properly outfitted to meet those requirements.

Let me just briefly remind you of the three keys to increased health:

Supplementation—Your diet may be as riddled with holes as any traffic sign in small-town USA. Our foods, especially the over-processed variety so prevalent today, just don't provide us with the nutrients that we need. You must supplement your diet with a good multivitamin to get the benefits of the many nutrients your body needs not only to stay alive but for protection.

Good Diet—Perhaps no other factor will play a larger role in your health than good nutrition. If you are eating right, you'll help prevent many of the illnesses our society suffers from. You'll look and feel healthier, you'll maintain your weight, and you'll live longer—all by eating better.

Exercise—It's high time we stopped watching prime time and started living it. Instead of watching other people live exciting, fulfilling lives, we should be out there creating our own spectacular stories. Get involved in sports, start working out and by all means involve your children. You'll prevent disease, improve your chances of a longer, more productive life, and you'll build quality memories that you'll cherish forever.

Chapter Four

Prescription Refills R' Us

There's an old joke about a guy on his hands and knees crawling on the street. A police officer comes up and asks, "Hey, pal, what do you think you're doing?" The guy looks up and says, "I lost $20 on Mulberry Street, and I'm looking for it." The police officer scratches his head, and says, "But this is Maple Street." The guy responds, "I know. But the lighting is better on Maple Street."

When it comes to choosing between treating our maladies with prescription drugs or with natural methods, most of us are just like the guy on Maple Street. We take the easy way out and look for health-care solutions "where the lighting is better." Who cares if it's the wrong place?

The prescription drug companies don't mind. Our addiction—and it is an addiction—to prescription drugs is making the pharmaceutical industry billions. That's not to say that some of the drugs coming out of the pharma-pipeline aren't valuable and useful. They are—especially the ones that we need to treat trauma patients and other victims of injury or disease. I have many friends in the prescription drug industry and think that, in many cases, they do a bang-up job in helping people alleviate the pain and suffering of illness and disease.

By and large, we do have control over many of the risk factors associated with the modern disease process. Heart disease, diabetes and many forms of cancer head the list of physical ailments that are in many cases highly preventable—if we take the necessary steps to ward them off. But often we don't, reassured, somewhat, by the knowledge that there is a perfect little pill out there that will enable us to beat the condition.

FAST FACT:

Retail pharmacies filled three billion prescriptions in the U.S. in 2000.

THE COST OF DRUGS

We're throwing money away on many prescription drugs, and we don't even realize it. Take cholesterol-lowering drugs— millions already do—for example. According to a January 6, 2003, article in *Fortune magazine,* more than forty-four million Americans took the best-selling cholesterol prescription drug in 2002. It's slated to earn $10 billion annually for the company that makes it. That's an amazing number of people for a drug that's only six years old.

How financially successful are cholesterol-lowering drugs? The leading drug in that category earned about four times as much money as another widely touted wonder drug—Viagra. You can't blame the cholesterol prescription drug makers; they're in the business of capturing market opportunities. The fifty-two million Americans, who, according to the National Institute of Health, have cholesterol problems present the mother of all marketing opportunities. These folks love their little blue pills and especially the five million Americans who comprise what the Food and Drug Administration calls a "congestive heart failure epidemic."

Research, development, and FDA approval can take upward of ten years and cost in excess of a $100 million. Cholesterol lowering drugs don't solve high cholesterol—they simply lower your cholesterol levels. These drugs don't cure the condition; they just rein it in for awhile, providing a health alternative that we are willing to pay for. Where is the incentive to research a cure when setting up a lifetime of treatment floods the coffers with healthy profits from the not-so-healthy masses?

It's not just cholesterol cures that Americans crave. Apparently, our appetite for over-the-counter drugs matches our appetite for prescription drugs. According to a new study by the University of Michigan Health System published in the February 24, 2003, edition of *Archives of Internal Medicine,* the cost of treating the common cold to the U.S. economy is $40 billion a year. That's substantially more than other conditions such as asthma, heart failure, and emphysema. What's more, Americans can't seem to rid themselves of the notion that a miracle cure exists down at the drugstore or at the doctor's office.

"A cold is the most commonly occurring illness in humans, so it was no surprise that there are approximately 500 million colds each year in the U.S.," said A. Mark Fendrick, lead author of the study. "What was a surprise is how often the public uses the health-care system to treat a cold."

The study found that Americans spend $2.9 billion on over-the-counter drugs and another $400 million on prescription medicines for symptomatic relief. Additionally, more than $1.1 billion is spent annually on the estimated forty-one million antibiotic prescriptions for cold sufferers, even though antibiotics have no effect on a viral illness.

"We found that the common cold leads to more than 100 million physician visits annually at a conservative cost estimate of $7.7 billion per year," Fendrick said. "More than one-third of patients who saw a doctor received an antibiotic prescription. While these unnecessary costs are problematic, what is more concerning is how these treatment patterns contribute to the development of antibiotic resistance, a significant public health concern."

FAST FACT: License to Print Money

According to its 1999 annual ranking of America's most profitable industries, *Fortune magazine* found the pharmaceutical industry on top in its key benchmark categories: return on revenues, return on assets, and return on shareholders' equity. Another recent report, this one entitled "Profiting from Pain" from the research group Families USA, said that while working families pay more and more for prescription drugs, the pharmaceutical industry has been the most profitable U.S. industry for each of the past ten years.

DEPENDENCE ON PRESCRIPTION DRUGS

What we really need is a prescription drug that will wean us off prescription drugs. If we can't, that dependence is going to take us straight to the poorhouse.

In 2001, prescription drug spending increased 16.9 percent, according to the *2001 Express Scripts Drug Trend Report*. The average wholesale price cost was $592.05—an $85.42 increase above the 2000 figure of $506.63.

In the report, more than half the increase in total spending—56.8 percent—is attributable to a rise in per prescription costs due to higher prices and use of more expensive medications. Increased utilization accounted for 37.3 percent of the increase, while the introduction of new drugs in 2001 was responsible for 5.9 percent. In addition, for the fourth consecutive year, inflation in drug prices—at 5.5 percent in 2001—topped 5 percent. Price inflation accounted for 35 percent of the overall 2000-2001 drug-expenditure increase.

It's also apparent that we're spending most of our money on a small handful of drugs. According to the Express Scripts Report, about 50 cents of every dollar spent on prescription drugs went for drugs in just 10 of 99 therapeutic categories in 2001: Antihypertensives, antidepressants, antihyperlipidemics (cholesterol reducers), gastrointestinal drugs, antidiabetics, antirheumetics, antiasthmatics, antihistamines, calcium channel blockers, and dermatologicals.

"Antihyperlipidemics, the medicines used to treat high blood cholesterol, were the third most-used therapy class, after blood pressure and antidepressant drugs. In recent years, dramatic increases in the use of antihyperlipidemics have been spurred by evidence that their use reduces mortality, new guidelines that increase the total number of patients eligible for treatment and extensive direct-to-consumer advertising," said the report.

What better marketing ploy than to convince Americans that a given drug may well save their lives? And what better way to get that message across than to go over the heads of society's caregivers—the doctors, nurses, and other health-care professionals who treat Americans—and go right to consumers via televised advertisements?

THE MEDIUM IS THE MESSAGE

It's tough to watch a football game or situation comedy on the tube without an ad popping up with a smiling man or woman enjoying life thanks to the latest wonder drug. Defenseless against such a barrage, many Americans stop doubting whether the latest miracle drug may work for them and start making phone calls to their doctor's office to write up a prescription.

After all, the pharmaceutical industry isn't foolish. They spend millions on advertising because it works. Consider this study from the National Institute for Healthcare that claims spending on new, heavily advertised drugs pushed drug expenditures up 84 percent—or $42.7 billion—from 1993 through 1998. "More than 30 percent of that growth was the direct result of sales in four therapeutic categories—oral antihistamines, antidepressants, cholesterol reducers and anti-ulcerants—which tend to include heavily advertised drugs," the study reports. "In 1998, for every dollar spent by the U.S. pharmaceutical industry on R&D, nearly 50 cents was spent on product promotion."

THE COST OF LETTING US KNOW JUST HOW SICK WE ARE

Those of us who've spent some time in the health-care industry know that advertising isn't the only reason why prescription-drug costs are so high. The aging of our most populous demographic (the Baby Boomers), and the increased use of newer, more pricey prescription drugs have contributed to the bulging coffers of the pharmaceutical industry.

That said, there's little doubt that using television advertising to go over the heads of health-care provider's and straight to the American people was a stroke of genius from a revenue-generating point of view. Any student of Marketing 101 knows that the key to moving supply is to increase the demand for that supply.

According to NDCHealth, a New York City-based health-care information company, Americans paid about $208 billion in 2001 for prescription drugs —almost double that spent in 1996. Coincidentally—or perhaps not so coincidentally—the rate that prescription drug companies spent on marketing, defined by NDCHealth as consumer advertising and sales meetings with doctors, also rose. In 1999 alone, advertising spending by the pharmaceutical industry rose a staggering 234

Where the Rubber Meets the Road: Prescription Drug Costs and Advertising

A 1999 study from the National Institute of Healthcare maintains that the high cost and increased advertising of prescription drugs by the pharmaceutical industry are intertwined. Here are some highlights from the report:

- From 1993 to 1998, spending on heavily advertised drugs increased by 612 percent, spending on antidepressants increased 240 percent, spending on cholesterol-reducing drugs increased by 194 percent, and ad spending on anti-ulcerant drugs increased by 71 percent.

- The ten drugs most heavily advertised to consumers in 1998 accounted for 22 percent ($9.3 billion) of the total increase in retail-drug spending between 1993 and 1998.

- While generally under-advertised generic drugs accounted for 46 percent of all prescription units dispensed in 1998, they represent only 8 percent of all prescription drug sales.

- Increased spending is attributable to both the average price per prescription (with new drugs costing more than twice as much per prescription as older drugs—$71.49 compared to $30.46 in 1998) and the number of prescriptions filled (which grew from 1.9 billion in 1993 to 2.5 billion in 1998).

- Higher average prices per prescription accounted for about 64 percent of the five year increase in spending.

percent (although that number plummeted to just 19 percent in 2000). But all those marketing dollars worked like a charm. Americans bought into the notion pushed by Big Medicine that relief for any number of health ailments was just a perfect little pill away. "The pharmaceutical industry is a very healthy industry," said Sheldon Silverberg, a pharmaceutical-industry analyst at NDCHealth. "People are walking into doctors' offices after seeing commercials."

Given that Americans shelled out $208 billion for prescription-drugs in 2001, and that the pharmaceutical industry invested—and that's the right word for it—a grand total of $2.8 billion on consumer advertising (based on numbers from Quintiles Informatics, a consulting firm), that's an investment return that would have Warren Buffet dancing on the conference table.

According to Quintiles Informatics, the bulk of the prescription drug industry's marketing expenses go to pay their legions of sales representatives who call on doctors, nurses, hospitals, and managed care companies. Quintiles pegs the number of sales representatives in 2002 at 81,600, an increase of 45 percent since 1998. In addition, the pharmaceutical industry held 370,300 meetings and events for doctors last year designed to promote their prescription drugs—an increase of almost 18 percent. "Doctors continue to get the lion's share of the money spent to promote medicines," the company reports.

O.K., fair is fair. We live in a capitalist society that rewards those who take risks, and that's exactly what the pharmaceutical industry does every time it drops millions of dollars into prescription drug research with no guarantee that a nascent drug will ever pan out.

So it's only fair that when the industry does come up with a potential winner, it should get the chance to market the product to the fullest extent, just as Ford Motor Company does with cars and trucks and Proctor & Gamble does with soap and toothpaste. But, what if the ads that Big Medicine produces aren't entirely accurate? What if they leave some crucial information out or twist relevant information to distract or confuse the health-care consumer?

That's exactly what researchers at Dartmouth Medical School say a few in the pharmaceutical industry are doing in their product advertisements.

Dr. Steven Woloshin and Dr. Lisa Schwartz, both assistant professors, and H. Gilbert Welch, professor of medicine and of community and family medicine from Dartmouth Medical School and the Veterans Affairs Medical Center, released a study in October 2001 which highlights how consumers can be ill informed by prescription drug commercials.

The investigators assessed prescription-drug advertising in ten leading magazines. They included four women's magazines *(Family Circle, Ladies Home Journal, Better Homes & Gardens, Good Housekeeping)*, three men's magazines *(Sports Illustrated, Men's Health, Gentleman's Quarterly)* and three general population magazines *(Time, Newsweek, People)*.

"Consumers are increasingly exposed to direct-to-consumer advertisements for prescription products," Woloshin said. "In turn, physicians are increasingly confronted with patients who ask questions, or who make suggestions, on the basis of these advertisements.

"Our findings indicate that these advertisements rarely quantify a medication's expected benefit and instead make an emotional appeal. This strategy probably leaves many readers with the perception that the drug's benefit is large, and that everyone who uses the drug will enjoy the benefit. The provision of complete information about benefit would serve the interests of physicians and the public."

Woloshin's staff examined seven issues of each title published between July 1998 and July 1999. They documented sixty-seven advertisements that appeared a total of 211 times during the study and were more often placed in magazines predominantly read by women. Of these, 133 (63 percent) were for drugs to alleviate symptoms, fifty-four (26 percent) to treat disease and twenty-three (11 percent) to prevent illness. "In the sixty-seven different advertisements, promotional techniques used included emotional appeals (67 percent) and encouragement of consumers to consider medical causes for their experiences (39 percent)," the study reported. "Nearly 90 percent of advertisements described the benefit of medication in vague, qualitative terms rather than with data, however, half the advertisements used data to describe infrequent side effects. And no advertisements mentioned cost."

And it's not just Dartmouth Medical School. Uncle Sam, too, has checked in with some doubts about the accuracy of the pharmaceutical industry's prescription-drug advertisements. According to a December 2002 report from the U.S. General Accounting Office, some companies "have repeatedly disseminated misleading advertisements for prescription drugs even after being cited for violations, and millions of people see the deceptive commercials before the government tries to halt them."

The report caught the attention of some powerful people in Washington. "The evidence suggests that consumers are paying a lot of attention to these ads, so it's imperative that they be accurate," said Senator Susan Collins, a Maine Republican. "If the increase in utilization is based on false claims, that's very troubling."

Federal rules generated by the Department of Health and Human Services (HHS) say drug ads must present a fair, accurate account of both benefits and risks. From August 1997 to August 2001, the agency issued eighty-eight letters accusing drug companies of advertising violations—forty-four for broadcast advertisements, thirty-five for print ads, and nine that cited both types of ads.

In most cases, the agency said, companies overstated the effectiveness or minimized the risks of medicines. In 2000, for example, HHS forced one prominent company to stop airing certain commercials for its osteoporosis drug Actonel after discovering that information about the drug's risks was obscured by "fast-paced, rapidly changing, distracting images" on the screen.

Certainly, media advertisements aren't all inaccurate. But enough are to raise some eyebrows in the health-care industry and in Washington. Big Medicine and Madison Avenue have combined to present an image of prescription drugs as wonder drugs that can turn unhealthy people's lives around. It's marketing masquerading as science.

Not only is such a practice flat out wrong, it's dangerous—dangerous to the millions of Americans who fall for the exaggerated claims coming out of prescription drug ads and who often don't get any relief from their ailments as a result. And, with increased demand as a direct result of the big media push by Big Medicine, the price of such wonder drugs will continue to go up and up, placing even more of a burden on our health-care industry.

How much more pressure can it take?

EVERYTHING OLD IS NEW AGAIN

Harvey MacKay, author of *Swim with the Sharks without Being Eaten Alive*, said that marketing is creating a condition that allows the buyer to convince himself to buy.

The pharmaceutical industry has done a great job of doing just that. Making people want something they otherwise can't have is an old marketing gambit. I remember a new restaurant I used to visit in L.A. that told people who called in for a reservation that they were all booked up—even though the restaurant was virtually empty! But people kept calling in greater numbers, convinced that a restaurant that busy was a hip and exciting place to go. The restaurant took off as a result.

Just good, basic marketing, right? But once you create a climate where a customer convinces himself to buy, just what, exactly, is he buying? In the prescription-drug market, the evidence suggests that the customer may not be buying what he thinks he's buying.

For example, consider the flood of "new" prescription drugs that are hitting the marketplace.

According to a May 2002 study by the U.S. Food and Drug Administration, two-thirds of the drugs approved from 1989 to 2000 were modified versions of existing drugs. Worse, some were even identical to those already on the market rather than truly new medicines. In the same report, the FDA said that most of the increased spending on new prescription drugs was on products that the agency had determined "did not provide significant benefits over those already on the market."

Some of those "reformulated" drugs were—surprise, surprise—among the prescription drugs that were most aggressively advertised, said the FDA. "The plain fact is that many new drugs are altered or slightly changed versions of existing drugs, and they may or may not be all that much better than what's already available," said Nancy Chockley, president of the National Institute for Healthcare Management Foundation, which wrote the report. "Consumers should be more aware of that."

Welcome to the "Me-Too" prescription drug culture. The FDA said that of the 1,035 drugs approved by the agency from 1989 to 2000, only 361, or 35 percent, contained new active ingredients. The rest contained active ingredients that were already available in other medicines on the market. Given that data, the study discovered that effective new medicines—those the agency describes as ones with new chemical ingredients that offer significant improvements over existing drugs—made up only 15 percent of those approved.

Some say Wall Street is to blame for such a profits-at-any cost culture that currently permeates the prescription drug industry. To keep stock prices up high where investors like them, a pharmaceutical company has to keep making profits come hell or high water. "Me-too" drugs are a great way to do that. In the FDA study, drug companies were increasingly relying on the "Me-too" products as patents on top-selling drugs expired and truly new medicines that could increase revenue were not being discovered as fast as investors expected. Cheaper to make, reformatted drugs also provide a high return on investment, as making them is much less expensive and less time-consuming than trying to find a new medicine. "This is more evidence that the pharmaceutical companies are turning more into marketing companies," Chockley said.

The FDA concluded its study on reformatted drugs by saying the pharmaceutical industry is no different than any other industry in marketing "new and improved" products. Using Proctor & Gamble and it's popular "Tide" washing detergent as an example, the report suggests that the prescription-drug industry "has learned" to be like the Proctor & Gambles of the world—putting a new spin on old products.

FAST FACT: Older, Bolder and Pricier

The U.S. Food and Drug Administration said that while reformatted prescription drugs don't improve on their predecessors, that doesn't stop the pharmaceutical industry from charging more for them.

In 2000, the average price of a modified drug not given a priority review by the FDA was about $65—almost double the price of a drug approved before 1995, the study said.

DOCTOR, GIVE ME THE (STRAIGHT) NEWS

In the June 2003 issue of Reader's Digest a reader submitted the following experience:

> *Our nephew was getting married to a doctor's daughter. At the wedding reception, the father of the bride stood to read his toast, which he had scribbled on a piece of scrap paper. Several times during his speech, he halted, overcome with what I thought was a moment of deep emotion. But after a particularly long pause, he explained, 'I'm sorry. I can't seem to make out what I've written down.'*
>
> *Looking out into the audience, he asked, 'Is there a pharmacist in the house?'*

There's no doubt that doctors can scribble out prescriptions. One topic where health-care industry observers tread lightly is the touchy subject of doctors lining their pockets with kickbacks and perks from the prescription-drug industry to tout specific drugs to patients.

American consumers spent over $200 billion on prescription drugs in 2001, more than double what the nation spent on drugs in 1996. How much of that, if any, is attributable to doctors recommending the prescription drugs that the industry wants them to recommend?

Tough to say, but the speculation is out there. Is it what some in the health-care profession call "legalized bribery?" How are the army of sales reps hired by the pharmaceutical industry influencing, if at all, the prescription drug decisions of doctors and other care givers?

The pharmaceutical sales rep/doctor relationship is a strange one even for this industry. Unlike most industries, which target consumers directly, the pharmaceutical industry targets the middleman—in this case the doctor. As has already been alluded to, the industry is also, at the same time, going over the heads of doctors with commercial pitches touting the latest miracle drug. By working the doctor angle too, the pharmaceutical industry is covering its bases by persuading doctors to prescribe their prescription drugs to patients. In 2001, the industry spent almost $9.4 billion on marketing to U.S. doctors, according to Verispan, a market-research firm. So there's definitely some "influencing" going on. No arguing that.

But how far are they going? *The New York Times* recently reported that in one case police raided the overseas offices of one American prescription drug company. When the dust cleared, forty staff and thirty doctors were under investigation for what the locals called "comparaggio"—prescribing drugs in exchange for gifts, such as laptop computers and expensive vacations. Other cases where sales reps have given personal digital assistants to doctors and invited them on "consulting trips" to exotic locales are commonplace. Some funny business is going on. Otherwise, why has the number of pharmaceutical sales reps doubled since 1995 even though the number of doctors in the U.S. has stayed pretty much the same?

While few can say for sure just how prevalent the issue of "legalized bribery" has beset the health-care industry, it's an albatross around the neck of reputable doctors everywhere who have to deal with it. If patients can't trust their family doctor to make sure they're getting the right treatment—or getting no prescription drug treatment unless it's really needed—then the underpinnings of the health-care industry are really beginning to wobble.

It's one thing for the prescription drug industry to make billions off of potentially deceptive advertising. It's quite another to interfere with the doctor-patient relationship. In the end, that's where the foundation for our health system rests—for better or for worse.

FAST FACT: Killer Drugs?

Prescription drugs are the fourth-leading cause of death. The first three are: heart attacks, cancer and strokes.

Source: Mercola.com

A SUCCESS STORY

Forever dependent on one prescription drug or another to help ease the pain from various illnesses, Rita Joy finally got sick and tired of it.

Overweight by forty pounds and constantly tired and dragging her feet, particularly after taking some allergy drugs that made her want to take a nap more than anything else, Rita changed her life around by cutting fatty meats and salty snacks out of her diet. She also began a walking program down at the YMCA.

To augment those changes in her life, Rita also began taking doses of vitamin C and vitamin E to help build up her immune system against the persistent colds and flues that plagued her life.

Today, Rita easily slips into a size four and has gotten off the prescription-drug roller coaster for good. Using a sophisticated blend of vitamins, minerals and herbal ingredients, Rita has boosted her metabolism, decreased her appetite, reduced food cravings and increased her energy levels.

And now those little brown prescription-drug bottles are a thing of the past.

Chapter Five

Healthy Habits

Disney's classic *Bambi* taught a number of wonderful principles. While eating clover blossoms isn't what we would call delightful, to Thumper and his siblings they represented an easy and better-tasting alternative to the "greens." When Bambi arrives on the scene, Thumper is quick to invite him to their feast in the meadow. Bambi, not knowing any better, takes a big mouthful of greens. With a laugh, Thumper explains that there is a better way. And just as Thumper is about to engulf the delicious blossom, his mom asks, "Thumper, what did your father tell you about eating the blossoms and leaving the greens?" Thumper then stands at attention and recites:

> *"Eating greens is a special treat.*
> *It makes long ears and great big feet.*
> *But it sure is awful stuff to eat."*

Thumper quickly pulled from memory a family motto that set his "foraging" behavior back in line. Our children watch and model our behaviors. Yes, the greens sure can be "awful stuff to eat," but so was doing homework, weeding the garden, and taking the garbage out. Our children must be taught from their own dinner tables the long-term value of good nutrition. Parents can create an environment where eating healthy and keeping a clean room stand on equal footings. Pushing aside the vegetables and not doing assigned chores can be treated the same way. Nutritional procrastination carries a price. Thumper is more than the cute rabbit; he can now play a new role in our homes as the spokesperson for better family nutrition.

THE HARDEST STEP TO TAKE IS THE FIRST

By gradually adding a few good habits while working to drop a few bad ones, you'll make changes in your life that will delay the arrival of old age and death. My twin brother charted a one-year course by making a commitment to his new and improved self, "Future Charlie." As "Historical Charlie," he had a vision of where he wanted to end up and started with the end in mind. With little expense, he strategically placed his promises to "Future Charlie" on 3X5 cards where he could be constantly reminded of his commitments. Charlie promised himself that he would exercise every day, eat a good diet, reduce his portion sizes and use supplements to ensure better health. He took a path previously not taken and "that has made all the difference." After a year of reading—and keeping—these promises everyday, "Historical Charlie" reached his goals. It wasn't the gym membership or the best-selling book on the latest dieting techniques that did it. Charlie forged a new set of habits and set out on a path with the intent of finding his optimal physiological self.

Robert Frost's popular poem, "The Road Not Taken" paints a powerful visual that aptly fits this challenge. Some might well be on their way down the unworn path to wellness and prevention. They can read the poem and already say that it has made all the difference.

The Road Not Taken

Two roads diverged in a yellow wood,
And sorry I could not travel both
And be one traveler, long I stood
And looked down one as far as I could
To where it bent in the undergrowth;
Then took the other, as just as fair,
And having perhaps the better claim,
Because it was grassy and wanted wear;
Though as for that the passing there
Had worn them really about the same,
And both that morning equally lay
In leaves no step had trodden black
Oh, I kept the first for another day!
Yet knowing how way leads on to way,
I doubted if I should ever come back.
I shall be telling this with a sigh
Somewhere ages and ages hence:
Two roads diverged in a wood, and I-
I took the one less traveled by,
And that has made all the difference.

WHAT ABOUT BOB?

Let me tell you about Bob, who intentionally doesn't want his last name to be shared because he's still ashamed at how much he weighed before he took control of his weight and his life.

Bob retired from law enforcement in 1994. When he retired he was in pretty good shape. But once he was no longer on the force, he let everything go. He lost interest in working out and in staying fit. He didn't get enough sleep. He didn't eat the right kinds of foods. And, like most of us, he was under a lot of stress from a new job. He ballooned up to 604 pounds, and he thought he just couldn't change. He tried a few different diets and found they didn't work. Then he went to a health website and got some ideas about weight loss—some of them new ideas.

He started walking first, then doing light weights. His workout increased to four times a week, and he started feeling better. He began to sleep better. He gained a new determination to continue.

Now he has a full workout weight gym in his basement, and he continues to work out at least four days a week and is on his treadmill at least three days a week. When he can, he takes walks during his lunch break.

At the same time he started exercising, he began eating the right foods and watching his fat and sugar intake. He also takes dietary supplements in the form of protein, vitamins, and minerals. Compared to a year ago, he looks, feels, and acts like a new person.

GOAL SETTING

Goal setting can be a tricky business. Often, especially when it comes to advancing our health, we set our goals too high. Consider New Year's resolutions. We all make them, right? But often we say we want to lose 20 pounds by Valentine's Day or train to run the Boston Marathon in April. Grand goals? Yes. Realistic goals? No.

So instead of saying, "I want to lose 40 pounds by the time summer rolls around," take a more measured approach. Say, "I'm going to take healthy steps to lose weight and keep at it. By the time summer rolls around, I know I will feel better and look better if I just stick to my new health regimen." You will find that by simply starting a health program that includes a quality supplement, a better diet and consistent exercise, you will see results. You will lose weight, you will get sick less often, and you will avoid unnecessary visits to the treatment centers. While we are all different in body shape and size, we stand equal when it comes to the benefits available from a healthier lifestyle.

THREE GOAL ZONES

Perhaps you've already noticed, but in the two stories I've shared with you—about Charlie and Bob—there were three things that they added to their life to make spectacular health changes. In fact, Chapter Three is dedicated to these three areas. Let me just briefly talk about them again here.

Supplementation—Perhaps the easiest route to improved health is through the addition of a quality multi-vitamin and mineral supplement. A daily multi-vitamin regimen can ensure that your body gets not only the nutrients it needs to survive, but also in the amounts that it needs to protect itself from environmental risk factors. Find a quality supplement—the single-serve packets you find on the counters of convenience stores will not cut it. Look for a company with solid scientific backing, a good quality assurance program, and a reputation for producing the best product around. Keep in mind that pharmacists went to school to learn about drugs, and doctors were trained to treat. While their input is valuable, it should be balanced by your own personal qualitative efforts.

Good Diet Habits—If supplementation is the easiest change, then making good diet changes and choices is probably the most important. Start giving vegetables the starring role in your eating habits. Cut back on sugar, fats,

75

and processed foods. Eat more fresh foods like fruits and vegetables and try to eat more fowl and fish than red meat.

The great thing about making diet changes is that they can be very small yet make great differences. Instead of the standard white bread, switch to whole-grain breads. Instead of the processed "fruit" products, get the real thing. Add a rule to always eat your veggies first. Start drinking more water. Tiny changes in your diet can be easy, yet they will make a big difference.

Exercise—It's hard to make the time and find the energy and even desire to get up off of the sofa—especially if a favorite show is on—and get moving. Exercise can be equated with any physical activity. As long as you're "up and doing," you'll make a difference. Gardening, cleaning the house, going for a walk, playing basketball with the kids or going for a swim all count as good physical activity. And remember that we're talking about thirty minutes of cumulative activity throughout the day. While not always convenient, I try to take a hike everyday. Why? Well, I do it for my kids. I believe if I can sacrifice a little bit now, I can stay around a little longer later. I look at exercise as a critical component to my retirement strategy. What good is a stable retirement fund without the health to enjoy it?

Starting out, keep in mind that it usually takes at least four to six weeks before you'll even notice a physical change. That's completely normal. Don't get discouraged when at the end of week one your weight hasn't changed. If you're making these positive changes, then something good is happening—I promise.

Think of it like this: If you start taking a cardiovascular supplement like vitamin E, you won't wake up one morning and say, "Hmm, my LDL's sure do feel better today." You just can't feel something like that. So you've got to keep plugging away at it. Trust in the science that backs up these health practices. You may not see the results until your next physical—but trust that those changes are happening.

There's an old saying that it takes thirty days to build a good habit and thirty seconds to break it while bad habits take only thirty seconds to form and thirty days to break. So many people shoot themselves in the foot by stopping their programs just when change is about to happen. Don't give up on it. Too many of the good changes aren't visible to the naked eye—but they will become apparent, say fifty years from now, when you're outliving all of your friends or just out living with your friends.

Who Am I?

"I am your constant companion; I am your greatest helper or heaviest burden. I will push you onward or drag you down to failure. I am completely at your command. Half the things you do might just as well turn over to me, and I will be able to do them quickly and correctly. I am easily managed—you must merely be firm with me. Show me exactly how you want something done and after a few lessons, I will do it automatically. I am the servant of all great people, and alas, of all failures as well. Those who are great, I have made great. Those who are failures, I have made failures. I am not a machine, though I work with all the precision of a machine plus the intelligence of a human. You may run me for a profit or run me for ruin—it makes no difference to me. Take me, train me, be firm with me. And I will place the world at your feet. Be easy with me, and I will destroy you. WHO AM I? I AM HABIT."

—Unknown

TEN KEYS TO HEALTHY HABITS

There are no silver bullets. Losing weight and preventing chronic illness won't happen in the emergency room. Closing the gap between your current status and your optimum biological potential lies in development of good habits. Best-selling author Og Mandino summed it best, "In truth, the only difference between those who have failed and those who have succeeded lies in the difference of their habits. Good habits are the key to all success. Bad habits are the unlocked door to failure. Thus, the first law I will obey, which precedes all others, is—'I will form good habits and become their slaves.'"

1. Give It a Shot.

I recall an anecdote from an interview with Hall of Fame hockey legend Wayne Gretzky. He said in his early days a coach made a great impression on him regarding the necessity of taking action. The words used by the coach to make his point? "You miss 100 percent of the shots you never take." Exactly. You miss 100 percent of the shots you never take.

Often, action means just taking something one step further than others. George Westinghouse, founder of the company that bears his name, once said that others in his day knew as much as he did about railroads, electricity and natural gas. But he took the action step. He invented the airbrakes to make trains safer, other devices to transmit gas and alternate current at a lower cost.

Former President of Chrysler Lee Iacocca said, "People say to me: 'You are a roaring success. How did you do it?' I go back to what my parents told me. Apply yourself. Get all the education you can, but then, by God, do something. Don't just stand there, make something happen."

These are the ideals by which you can begin to change your life. In my case, I use them to inspire and motivate me to continue to make the choices that make me healthier.

2. Create an Action Plan.

The secret to any lifetime endeavor is to have a plan, and every good plan should have short-term steps. Remember the old saying, "Yard by yard, life is hard, but inch by inch, life is a cinch." That's a good yardstick to go by when planning the kind of lifestyle and health-style changes you're going to make. We've already looked at how you can start with simple, little changes, so now it's up to you to decide on what those tiny alterations will be.

3. Mark the Start.

To get healthier, it's important to start off with a frame of reference as to how healthy you are right now. That will give you a benchmark to measure your progress against later on when you've started your own personal-wellness program.

I encourage you to take this self-health test from the U.S. Surgeon General. Add up your points in the end to see where you stand:

BENCHMARK

0 = No, never, or hardly ever
1 = Occasionally or rarely
2 = Sometimes or maybe
3 = Often
4 = Yes, or always

_____ I pay attention to the quality and amount of the foods I eat.
_____ I avoid fast foods and greasy, overcooked meals.

79

_____ I think my diet is well balanced and wholesome.

_____ I am aware that I feel different when I eat different foods, and I can choose foods that help me feel good.

_____ I minimize snacks and do not eat sugary or high-fat foods between meals.

_____ I drink fewer than 3 alcoholic beverages per week.

_____ I add little or no salt to my food.

_____ I eat at least 2 raw fruits or vegetables each day.

_____ I can tell the difference between my "stomach hunger" and "mouth hunger," and I don't eat when I am experiencing only "mouth hunger."

_____ It takes me 20 to 30 minutes to eat a meal.

_____ I feel good about how I eat and avoid using food as a reward, escape or punishment.

_____ I eat only small amounts of sweets or sugary things.

Finished? Add up your score and divide the total by 12.

Above 3:
You have good dietary habits and are at a decreased risk for some chronic diseases. Keep up the good work!

2 to 2.9:
You are average in your approach to eating. There are some areas that you can improve to feel better and be healthier.

1 to 1.9:
You do not have a healthy diet, but you do try. Look at the guidelines and pick one you would like to improve.

Below 1:
The good news is that there is a lot of room for improvement. Get help from your doctor or other treatment team members to change your eating habits.

4. Be Patient.

Rome wasn't built in a day and neither was Syracuse. So be patient. You're not going to literally see the fat melting off of your body. I'll wager that you didn't see it coming on either. But, if you keep with your program, you will see the day when you wake up and wonder where the fat went. That's why the next suggestion is so important.

5. Track Your Progress.

Start using a personal diary or a journal to chart your progress. That gives you a real-world look at how you're doing in your new diet or in your new exercise program. When you meet explicit goals—running a 5K or not eating red meat for thirty days—check it off. Then go ahead and create some new goals to work on. Once you get going and start feeling better, it becomes much easier to build up momentum. A diary is a great way for tracking that momentum. One trick I've played on myself over the years to adhere to a healthier diet is to place Post-it® notes or index cards around the house and around my workplace reminding me how much progress I'm making by eating fruits and vegetables. Over the years I've found that a little reminding goes a long way. If you really want to get vicious with yourself, tape an old picture of you when you weighed more on the refrigerator door.

Another great idea is to write down a description of how you feel and look before you start your program. Describe in detail both the good and bad of your life—your energy level, desire, self-esteem, illness frequency and so forth. You might even take a picture or measurements. Then keep that description. Look at it after six months of being on your program. You'll be surprised at the difference. And parents, this is a great way to see what the effects are on your kids. You might feel like a lab scientist observing rats and constantly taking notes, but you'll be impressed by the changes you see.

6. Be Creative.

The road to wellness need not be too strict or too regimented. It's a lot more fun and productive if you get a little creative along the way. For instance, I wanted to spend more time with my children—but I wanted to work out at the same time. So I'd organize bike rides and basketball games to keep me active and keep me engaged with my kids. It works in the kitchen, too. Why not get the whole family involved in making homemade fruit roll-ups or preparing a well-balanced meal? Remember, the object here isn't to deny you and your family the cornucopia of life. It's to enjoy it in a way that promotes longevity and vitality.

7. Expect Setbacks.

The famous educator John Condry once said, "Setbacks lead to innovation and renewed achievement." After all, the danger is not in the fall, as another saying goes, it's in failing to rise.

You will endure some failures and setbacks along your journey to wellness. That's O.K. Expect them. I remember when I first began jogging. Four weeks into my program I was running a mile a day easily. Then my business schedule picked up and I found myself traveling more and more and running less and less. A little confused and a lot frustrated, I started to see my progress slip a bit. After awhile, though, I picked myself up by bringing my gym bag and running shoes along with me to different cities. I found myself thrilled at the sites I saw running through great cities like Chicago and San Francisco. In the end, I turned a barrier into a joyful activity.

8. Get Your Rest.

Sleep is a critical part of maintaining good health. Just like developing a better diet and exercising, getting a good night's sleep is imperative to good health. I know that getting your rest is tough these days when many of us have to be up at the crack of dawn to get ready for work and the family ready as well. But foregoing sleep is a bad idea. It will just slow you down, negatively impact your productivity at home and in the workplace, and give you less energy to focus on a good diet and exercise program. So try and keep regular hours, even on Friday and Saturday night. Develop good, sleep-inducing habits, like reading to help you drift off to La-La Land. A good exercise regimen will help you sleep better as will cutting down on stimulants like caffeine and depressants like alcohol (which make you feel even more tired when you wake up).

9. Find a Network

A support network is a great idea when you're just starting out. If you're quitting smoking, for example, your local hospital or health clinic likely has a support group for ex-smokers. There is power in numbers, right? Or, if you want to start running, check with your local YMCA. Many have runner's groups for beginners, mid-level runners and experts. They're cheap to join and offer a wealth of benefits by joining up with others. I guarantee you'll make some new friends along the way, too.

And don't underestimate the power of accountability. I find it so much easier to get to the gym or to go for that run when I know that someone is counting on me to show up. It's easy to let ourselves down, but it hurts just a little bit more when we know that we let down a friend. Find a workout buddy—like a friend with similar goals, a spouse, or even your child—and then commit to each other to getting through the program together.

10. Include Your Physician.

If you're going to embark on a new diet or to hit the gym and take that rowing class, you should let your doctor know ahead of time. An annual comprehensive physical provides you with a thorough benchmark and will always be a recommended practice. Go back to your diary and write your weight down. Include the kinds of prescription drugs you're taking and the variety and frequency of flu and colds you've been getting. In six months, if you've been adhering to your new diet and fitness regime, check your journal entry from your last doctor visit and see how much weight you have lost and notice how infrequently you've been getting sick. Then smile and reward yourself for all the progress you've made.

Chapter Six

The Treatment Mentality

A touch of levity:

God populated the earth with vegetables of all kinds so that Man would live a long and healthy life.
And Satan created the ninety-nine cent double cheeseburger. And Satan said to Man, "Want fries with that?" And Man said, "Supersize them!"

And God created healthful yogurt, and Satan froze the yogurt and brought forth chocolate, nuts, and brightly colored candy to put on top. And Man gained more pounds.

And God brought forth running shoes, and Man resolved to lose those extra pounds.
And Satan brought forth cable TV, remote control, and potato chips. And Man clutched his remote and ate his chips. Satan saw this and said, "It is good."

And Man went into cardiac arrest. And God sighed and created quadruple bypass surgery.
And Satan created HMOs...

Source: Reader's Digest, March 2003

My desire to enter into the wellness-and-prevention market was fueled by an event that occurred about three years ago. My consulting firm works with pharmacology and biotechnology firms to help them identify and launch medical and treatment technologies. One of my clients is a not-for-profit research organization that is owned by a large health system. During one of my visits, I sat down with a group of physicians and researchers to identify a new working project that would align with their exempt purpose and charter of trying to help people.

We all agreed that one of the most preventable disease processes was diabetes, and that it can be treated through diet and exercise better than any other disease. We set out to develop a program that pro-actively screened a patient's blood sugar, while also addressing proper diet and nutrition practices. In short, we remodeled the status quo of intervention with a heightened sense of early detection and doing the right things in terms of managing the disease process of diabetes. Our team created a program that truly set out with the express intent of helping people live better, healthier lives.

When we pitched this program to the hospital administrators, to our surprise they had no interest in it. I will never forget the impact of the proverbial body blow when they explained that the hospital didn't get paid for not admitting patients. Our research project, while in alignment with the "charter," threatened to slow down the money spigot. The business of medicine and treatment, stockholders, mutual funds and Wall Street fashioned a model focused more on the bottom line than the Hippocratic Oath. Shortly thereafter, I made a conscience decision to disassociate myself with systems that were designed to profit by allowing people to develop advanced aspects of their disease process.

In real estate, the three most important words are location, location, location. Conversely, in health care the three most important words are admit, admit, admit. Doctors earn their keep by treating. Doctors get paid to prescribe medicines. Unfortunately, the system actually punishes doctors for spending time counseling patients on nutrition and diet. The billing process in health care is governed by reimbursement codes. These multi-digit numbers assign a procedure to a pre-determined fee. They simply organize and establish how the doctor will get paid for the services rendered. For example, if somebody comes into a doctor's office, and is overweight and living an obviously sedentary lifestyle, there is no question that the best service the doctor can provide is counsel in the direction of prevention and wellness. Unfortunately, the third-party providers—Medicare, Medicaid and the insurance companies—reward doctors for treating, testing, and surgically intervening. In fact, the system financially punishes doctors for taking time to offer assistance and getting these people back on the road to better health.

BARRIERS PLACED BY BIG MEDICINE

The health-care cost problem isn't strictly attributable to the hundreds of thousands of medical health practitioners across America. Doctors, nurses, emergency medical technicians, and the army of administrators and staffers at health-care companies and hospitals are doing commendable work in trying to keep up with the increasing demand for medical treatment. It's a fact of life that we are mortal and our bodies are not perfect. From premature babies to burn centers, from Alzheimer's to emergency room visits, there will always be someone who needs treatment.

The pharmaceutical companies are working overtime as well to deliver new prescription drugs to alleviate the pain Americans suffer. And the drugs the industry has developed to help expectant mothers, victims of accidents and violent crime, and other people who are in pain for no fault of their own are a Godsend.

The problem doesn't lie in these venues. Instead, it can be laid on the doorstep of the portions of the medical-industrial complex that are placing profits before prevention and the people who know in their heart of hearts that treatment is a poor substitute for precaution but still plow ahead with their plans for the next obesity wonder drug or perfect little pill to deal with the onslaught of heart disease.

This "treatment-first" mentality has resulted in a health-care system that doesn't promote better health—it promotes the treatment of ill health. It's a classic case of closing the barn door after the horse has escaped, and Americans are paying for it in more ways than one.

An August 26, 2002, issue of *Business Week* magazine stated, "The consequences of this shift of resources will be enormous for companies, workers and the government. It will mean a massive transfer of the nation's income, including profits, wages and tax dollars, to disease-oriented traditional medical care."

The article goes on to estimate that, "Perhaps one-third of all medical spending—some $600 billion dollars—may be unnecessary, out-of-date or even dangerous treatments."

BIG MEDICINE AS ENABLER

I once spoke with a good friend of mine who is a family-practice doctor. He lives in my town, and he knows I'm involved in prevention and wellness. He too is a believer in prevention, and he called to tell me that one of the national academies had just published a document called, "Health Prevention." I thought, "Wow! Finally the medical industry has understood the importance of prevention within the disease process."

I opened the "Health Prevention" manual excitedly. I soon realized, however, that the writers' idea of prevention was using tests to see if someone had a disease. That's it. The concept of going out and trying to prevent the disease process from occurring doesn't show up once in the manual. Here were thirty-six pages, which would be going out to virtually all family practice physicians entirely centered on how to test for prostate cancer and so forth. Not one word about disease prevention, just test intervention.

It all comes back to conventional wisdom. The industry has taken Herculean measures to convince us that health care is a back-end and not a front-end problem. It's a strategy that Dr. Tim O'Shea, author of *The Sanctity of Human Blood*, calls, "The Doors of Perception." O'Shea argues that from a health-care standpoint, conventional wisdom that finds mass acceptance is usually the result of manipulation of somebody with deep pockets and a hidden agenda. In the health-care sector, his examples of conventional wisdom gone wrong include:

- Pharmaceuticals restore health.
- Vaccination brings immunity.
- The cure for cancer is just around the corner.
- When a child is sick, he needs immediate antibiotics.
- When a child has a fever, he needs Tylenol.
- Hospitals are safe and clean.
- America has the best health care in the world.

O'Shea takes the pharmaceutical industry to task for the negative impact of such messages, taking special aim at the marketing end of the industry. "The drug companies are having their heyday now. They are not stupid by any stretch of the imagination. They have hired some of the most effective marketing people in the country to promote their products . . . the increased media exposure through direct advertisements on television to consumers is making a huge impact. However folks, the emperor has no clothes, and the emperor knows it. The traditional paradigm is fatally flawed. The drug/surgery model is an unmitigated disaster that has greatly contributed to pharmaceutical profits at the expense of the health of our country."

Strong stuff, but entirely on the mark.

THE HIGH COST OF HOSPITAL STAYS

The high cost of health care is not only forcing more Americans off the health-care plan rolls, it is also taking root in our nation's hospitals. While the average hospital charge for treating a patient admitted for a heart attack increased by one-third from 1993 to 2000, the length of patient stays was significantly reduced, according to the Agency for Healthcare Research and Quality (AHRQ).

According to the AHRQ, the total average charge for treating a heart-attack patient rose from $20,578 in 1993 to $28,663 in 2000. During the same period, the average number of days a patient spent in the hospital fell by 26 percent—from 7.4 days to 5.5 days. The total average charge is what hospitals charge for services, such as nursing care, laboratory analyses, diagnostic tests, medications, and use of operating rooms and patient rooms but not physicians' fees. Average total charges for many other high-cost conditions also increased between 1993 and 2000, while the time patients spent in the hospital decreased, according to AHRQ.

The agency also said that new technologies and rising medication costs explain much of the increase in average hospital charges. Even so, economic pressures have contributed to shortening the average patient stay for most conditions.

Other conditions for which charges have increased and patient stays have decreased are:

- **Blood poisoning (septicemia)**—from $17,909 to $24,365. The average hospital stay declined from 10.0 days to 8.2 days.
- **Heart rhythm disturbances (cardiac dysrhythmias)**—from $10,152 to $14,213. Average hospital stays declined from 4.7 days to 3.6 days.
- **Stroke (acute cerebral vascular disease)**—from $15,365 to $19,956. Average hospital stays fell from 9.5 days to 6.7 days.
- **Diabetes**—from $11,021 to $14,779. Average hospital stays declined from 7.4 days to 5.6 days.
- **Pneumonia**—from $12,860 to $15,104. Average hospital stays decreased from 7.8 days to 6 days.
- **Congestive heart failure**—from $11,995 to $15,293. Average hospital stays declined from 7.4 days to 5.6 days.
- **Nonspecific chest pain**—from $5,135 to $7,543. Average hospital stays fell from 2.5 days to 1.8 days.
- **Chronic obstructive lung diseases**—from $11,263 to $12,491. Average hospital stays declined from 7.2 days to 5.3 days.

Source: AHRQ, February 2003

FAST FACT: One in Five

One in five American families have at least one member who lacks medical coverage, putting the entire family at greater risk of poor health and financial ruin.

Source: The Institute of Medicine

WORST-CASE SCENARIOS

Potentially worse than the hospital-cost crisis is a reported trend among doctors that forces them to misrepresent their patients' needs to health-care providers in order to get the treatment they feel is needed.

In a May 2002 study by the University of Michigan Healthcare System, researchers found that some physicians are more willing to misrepresent patient information to avoid the "hassle factor" of the appeals process. Senior author of the paper Peter A. Ubel, M.D., said, "In an effort to control health-care costs, many insurance companies have developed mechanisms to limit physicians' ability to order expensive tests or treatments. If the HMO says 'no,' doctors can appeal, but often, it is a long and burdensome process. So in some cases, physicians lie about their patient's condition."

Using a random survey of 890 physicians with similar scenarios, the study found 11 percent of doctors said they would misrepresent the patient's condition to obtain HMO approval for surgery or additional procedures. Seventy-seven percent said they would appeal the decision, while 12 percent said they would accept it. But when hassle of the appeals process increased, so did the number of physicians willing to misrepresent patient information.

"The 'hassle factor' had a big influence over the doctors' actions," noted Ubel. "In fact, when physicians were told the appeal process would be 50 percent successful, 13 percent reported they would misrepresent, as opposed to 9 percent with a 95 percent success rate."

There isn't a sector within our communities that invests more personal time and money into their profession than doctors. Following the traditional four-year undergraduate, they toil another eight to ten years while building student loans that can easily surpass $250,000. Certainly a system that encumbers it's collective knowledge in the name of shareholder value has developed its own chronic weakness.

FAST FACT

According to *The Journal of the American Medical Association* and Dr. Barbara Starfield of the Johns Hopkins School of Hygiene and Public Health, the U.S. health-care system may contribute to poor health.

Annual Death Tolls from Medical Error (stemming from doctor error, manner, treatment or therapy):

- 12,000—unnecessary surgery.
- 7,000—medication errors in hospitals.
- 20,000—other errors in hospitals.
- 80,000—infections in hospitals.
- 106,000—non-error, negative effects of drugs.

At 225,000 deaths per year, doctor error constitutes one of the leading causes of death in the United States, said the JAMA article. Some of these deaths are attributable, the JAMA article said, to unnecessary treatment. Their analysis said that between 4 percent and 18 percent of consecutive patients experience negative effects in outpatient interactions, including:

- 116 million extra physician visits.
- 77 million extra prescriptions.
- 17 million emergency department visits.
- 8 million hospitalizations.
- 3 million long-term admissions.
- 199,000 additional deaths.
- $77 billion in extra costs.

THE END RESULT OF EXPENSIVE TREATMENT?

Hospital executives run their business no different than an auto dealership runs theirs. Cash flow keeps the lights on and the bills paid. The prevention philosophy and wellness programs are simply un-tested revenue models that appear financially pale in comparison to the vibrant treatment philosophy.

As a result of the medical-industrial complex's pro-treatment, anti-prevention health-care system philosophy, for the first time in almost a decade, health expenditures outpaced the growth of the U.S. economy. Spending rose 6.9 percent from 1999 to 2000 to $1.3 trillion, while the nation's gross domestic product (GDP) grew 6.5 percent. With the U.S. economy in a downward spiral, the federal government projected that health costs are likely to continue to grow faster than the GDP at least for the next few years.

This is a national tragedy. With a health-care system designed and built to treat the illness rather than create ways to prevent it from happening in the first place, we can only expect the high cost of health care in this country to continue to grow even higher. Why? Unhealthy lifestyle choices will continue to queue longer wait lines at these treatment facilities. America's health-care capacity—the number of available doctors, nurses, and technicians—is already stretched. As stated earlier, pharmaceutical companies simply earn a better return on their R&D by relieving symptoms not curing the conditions. Therefore, the treatment lines for you, your family, and employees never grows smaller. Simple economics will curtail demand by raising prices.

This equates to more Americans going without health care, more money for reduced hospital stays, and more combative stances between doctors and health-care organizations. And perhaps most damaging, the cost of being sick continues to fuel the economics of treatment.

We literally can't afford to allow this to happen. A transfer of resources to prevention in the form of wellness programs and preventive-care programs will alleviate most of this burden and stress that's currently placed on our health-care system, doctors, hospitals, and us.

Consequently, reforming our health-care system—and changing the way we look at health in this country—is not a luxury. It's a necessity.

CASE STUDY: Role Models from the Health-Care World

I think it's a myth that doctors want to see their patients as often as they can. Yes, that might bump up their income, but unhealthy patients tend to die quicker than their healthier counterparts. And that dries up income faster and longer than anything else.

Perhaps that's why more teaching hospitals and universities are starting to get on the prevention train and leaving their treatment programs back at the station. It's not happening as fast as I'd like it to, but it is definitely starting to happen.

Consider the Kirksville College of Osteopathic Medicine, a small rural teaching hospital in Missouri. There, the curriculum has changed from teaching students how to treat their patients when they are sick to showing them how to avoid getting sick in the first place. But Kirksville is, unfortunately, the exception rather than the rule. A recent study by the Science of Health Promotion reports that Kirksville has one of the most extensive and successful wellness programs among U.S. medical schools. But the study also points to the dearth of similar programs at U.S. teaching hospitals. Only 20 percent (32 of 141) of allopathic (M.D.) and osteopathic (D.O.) schools surveyed provide a health promotion program for students.

I think such programs will grow and grow, especially once medical colleges and universities realize how effective wellness programs are and see how positively Americans are responding to them. After all, the Kirksville program began way back in 1991, and it has taken twelve years for it to really take flight. Operating under the I-am-my-own-patient banner, the school's wellness program has been high and growing higher. In 1991, 41 of 290 eligible students voluntarily enrolled in the school's wellness program. Each year since, student involvement has increased, recently reaching a high point with 92 percent of the students voluntarily participating.

The program was so successful that Kirksville is now taking it on the road, bringing its mantra of wellness to schoolchildren across the U.S. In 2002, the school built a $650,000 science center exhibit called "The Healer Within," a 2,000-square-foot traveling exhibit that, among other educational programs, explains the preventive-concepts of health and wellness and is based on the principals of osteopathic medicine and self-directed wellness. It's a visually stimulating show (Why not? It's for kids!), where children are treated to a number of hands-on, colorful components. One program has students taking a virtual reality trip through the immune system where they become disease-fighting white blood cell warriors. Another has children gazing in wonderment as their nerves and muscles light up while doing mundane acts like turning a door handle or gripping a baseball. Another program features a cancer defender game that battles cancer by making healthy choices.

The Kirksville approach is the wave of the future for wellness programs, particularly for impressionable kids. It's no secret that the earlier you establish good lifestyle habits, the better. It's very difficult to get a forty year old to give up his cigarettes or Porterhouse steak dinners with all the trimmings.

Chapter Seven

Prevention Through Partnerships

The Center for Automotive Research reported that the "Big Three" automakers paid out roughly $8.8 billion in 2002 for health insurance for 2.2 million workers, retirees and dependents. According to a March 3, 2003, article in *Fortune* magazine, that estimate equates to an expense of roughly $1,200 per vehicle that rolls off the assembly lines for health care. The article goes on to state, "Health care, in fact, has become what hours and wages and job security were in the past—the make or break issue upon which unions and employers are increasingly giving no quarter. And that spells strike." The tension between corporate America and unions, small business and its employee base will grow in proportion to the extent that health premiums continue to outpace inflation.

Thirty years ago the expense of administering these benefit services to constituents and employees did not include the escalating price of treating a costly and largely preventable chronic-disease process. As the cost of treating cancer, heart disease, and diabetes as well as the incidence of these diseases continues to escalate, so too does the expense required by the government and corporate America.

As stated earlier, the challenge lawmakers and executive committees face is whether they can justify to their voters and shareholders coverage increases for illnesses that are predominantly driven by poor lifestyle habits. Employers cannot be held financially responsible for the gradual health risks associated with an abundance of drive-thru lunches and super-sized meal deals. Yet, employees are justifiably weary of benefit cuts when the media have shed new light on corporate greed, accounting shenanigans, and outrageous golden parachutes for the very executives that sign off on these cuts. Each side of this argument can easily find reasons to point a finger. Nevertheless, the solution to this divisive issue is not arduous collective bargaining sessions or debilitating strikes that ultimately punish not only the company and employees but also the end consumer.

Employer and employee working together, to collectively shift the focus to lifestyle habits that ultimately reduce health-care utilization will create tangible long-term benefits for both parties.

Benefits to Employers
- Reduced health-care costs.
- Reduced illness and injuries.
- Reduced absenteeism.
- Improved employee relations and morale.

Benefits to Employees
- Weight reduction.
- Reduced tension and feelings of stress.
- Improved well-being, enhanced self-image, and self-esteem.
- Improved physical function.

In the late '80s, it wasn't groundbreaking news at Union Pacific Railroad's headquarters that many of its 48,000 employees—predominantly middle-aged men—were overweight. At that time, UP's medical costs per employee were almost double the national average. So, in order to help workers improve their health and lose the extra weight, UP initiated a wellness program. This was no half-hearted effort either. In 2002 alone, UP invested $2 million dollars into the program, and their other efforts have won them several national health awards. CEO Dick Davidson explained this new emphasis as more than a good thing to do. "It became good business."

In 1987, UP opened an 8,000-square-foot gym at headquarters. Deals to give employees access to 450 gyms around the country soon followed. Dennis Richling, a staff physician at UP, was busy establishing other programs, like a peer-to-peer mentoring program for overweight employees. According to UP executives, their efforts are paying off to the tune of $50 million a year in medical-costs saving.

Yet for all the effort, the obesity rate at UP didn't drop, rather it increased. A 1995 survey showed that 40 percent of UP employees were obese (a number well above the national average of 15 percent). From 1995 to 2001, the percentage of obese employees rose from 40 percent to 52 percent. It's not for lack of trying on UP's part. The responsibility falls on the shoulders of the employees. No company can stop its employees from falling victim to the alluring temptation of fast food and other high-fat, high-calorie, low-nutrition snacks. And even with workout facilities being provided free of charge, no company can enforce attendance.

But, to UP's credit, they haven't given up yet. In 2002 they began referring some obese employees to an outside program that provides individual counseling and personalized weight-loss programs. Additionally, UP offered Meridia—a new, powerful weight-loss pill—to 150 obese employees free of charge. And finally, UP has begun to place fresh fruit in their headquarters to encourage healthy snacking.

Now that's a commitment to employee health and represents a noteworthy example for other companies to benchmark. The missing ingredient for Union Pacific involved a lethargic commitment level by its employees. Gym memberships and in-house gym equipment only work if the employee base makes a personal commitment to utilize the offering. Empowering a work environment that accepts and promotes healthy habits will quickly bridge the divisive gap of rising health-care premiums between employers and employees.

PREVENTIVE WELLNESS: THE KEY TO CUTTING DOWN THE COST OF BEING SICK

It's apparent each of us has the choice to lead a healthier life. But what is society (in general) and the health-care industry (in particular) doing to make such choices easier to make and to execute?

One way is the wellness-and-prevention program. Increasingly, hospitals, health-care providers, and even employers are turning to wellness programs designed to help us lead healthier lives. Once we do that, the business side of the health-care equation—the need to reduce the high cost of health care—will take care of itself.

Corporate wellness programs have gone way beyond the days when corporate America's idea of a healthy outing was a company softball game complete with kegs of beer and grilled hot dogs. Now, corporate wellness campaigns offer a vast menu of services geared toward helping employees embrace a healthy lifestyle. Such programs include massage therapy, smoking-cessation classes, stress-management meetings, diet and nutrition, and image consulting.

It's good business for companies to turn to wellness programs, too. They send a positive message to employees that management cares about them as individuals and wants to see them live healthier lives and prosper. Nothing wrong with that, right? The same goes for community-service organizations and health-care companies, who are also getting into the wellness game in a big way.

Consequently, officially organized wellness programs are popping up all over the societal landscape. Consider these examples:

- At Cuyahoga Community College near Cleveland, officials recently switched the school's onsite health-care emphasis from treatment to health promotion. Employees are encouraged to create a personal-wellness curriculum designed to meet individual needs. They chose from eighty-nine programs akin to college courses with credits and concentrations in social, intellectual, emotional, physical, spiritual, and occupational wellness. Employees can graduate with "honors" and a $100 bonus for completing the program. At the end of 2002, the college said that 35-40 percent of the college's full-time employees participate in the workplace wellness program.

- The New York State Department of Health and Managed Care Plans recently rolled out a program called "Move For Life!" A Joint Workplace Wellness Project. The project is designed to promote physical activity and healthy lifestyle choices in the workplace for New Yorkers. The program is an eight to ten week interactive class designed to encourage employees to make physical activity a part of their daily lives. The program rewards employees for participating, including certificates and prizes for participants achieving certain milestones throughout the program.

- At Georgetown University, employees "brown bag" it at weekly lunchtime health-care prevention seminars as part of the university's "Take a Flight into Health Wellness Series." The sessions, held every two weeks, provide faculty, staff and community members an opportunity to learn more about a wide variety of well-ness topics, including parenting, stress reduction, com-munication, physical health and workplace issues. Presenters are usually Georgetown University faculty or staff who share their expertise through presentations and question-and-answer sessions.

- At $30 per person, the Bank of America recently held a health-promotion program for retirees. The bank said that insurance claims were reduced an average of $164 per year for seminar participants.

- Coca Cola saw a decline in health-care claims, saving $500 per employee annually, for those who joined the company's HealthWorks fitness program.

- Prudential Insurance Company said that its health-care liability dropped from $574 to $312 for each employee enrolled in its corporate wellness program.

- A study, by The DuPont Corporation, of the effect of its comprehensive health-promotion program on absences among workers concludes that those involved with its wellness program had a 14 percent decline in disability days vs. 5.8 percent decline for employees who didn't take advantage of the program. Overall, the company saw 11,726 fewer net disability days.

WELLNESS IN THE WORKPLACE: AN INCUBATOR FOR PREVENTION

Successful corporate-wellness programs not only stem the exorbitant cost of treatment, they also boost company morale and employee retention. Additionally, healthy talent will look for and expect a result-oriented wellness partnership within their employment relationship. One good turn will lend itself to another. The upside of a vibrant and fit workforce is a consistent flow of healthy profits.

"Corporations now see health-management programs as the only long-term alternative to the continuing escalation of medical-care costs," noted D.W. Edington, director of the Health Management Research Center (HMRC) at the University of Michigan. "Nearly 60 percent of all companies and 95 percent of large companies have programs designed to encourage individuals to take some responsibility for their own health."

"There is greater return from investment in preventing healthy people from slipping into poor health behaviors than by trying to make chronically sick people well," he added. "Individuals benefit in terms of less pain and suffering and a higher quality of life. The corporation benefits in terms of less medical care costs and greater productivity."

According to a study by the HMRC, companies were first introduced to the concept of investing in health promotion programs in the 1970s. By the 1980s, employers were spending $5 per employee on workplace wellness programs and today they're shelling out $60 per employee for year-round programs that range from smoking cessation programs to lessons in warding off stress. The organization estimates the cost at about 1-2 percent of the typical medical care costs. Additional research from HMRC concludes that workplace wellness programs save employers $80 to $225 per employee per year in medical-care costs and an equal amount in productivity gains.

In doing so, wellness programs are reducing health-care costs in a number of ways, including:

- Providing healthier options other than doctor, hospital, and ER visits by giving wellness participants. tools and skills for self-care and self-responsibility.

- Motivating Americans to choose healthier lifestyles.
- Using health screenings to pinpoint high-health-risk Americans.
- Educating Americans on prevention of major illnesses.
- Reducing sick leave/absenteeism in the workplace.
- Improving productivity and reducing workers' compensation in the workplace.
- Introducing workers to dietary supplements that can help prevent disease.

Healthier people, lower health-care costs. What a concept! Those are the big reasons why wellness programs are one of the first big steps society can take to turn the tide against treatment and toward prevention. Such programs empower individuals within established peer groups to take a responsible approach to their own health and well-being by changing the focus of health-care services from treatment to prevention.

Health Care at the Top of Employee Benefits

In a 2000 study co-authored by World at Work and the Employee Benefit Research Institute, employees—by a wide margin—rate health care as their most important employee benefit.

In the study, 65 percent of workers view their health insurance benefits as most important and 17 percent rank health benefits as the second most important benefit. The study also said that increasingly the best and most affordable way to help workers with their health-care needs is through corporate wellness programs.

WAVE OF THE FUTURE

Corporate wellness programs look like they are here to stay. If companies can save money by showing workers how to live healthier lives and employees can use wellness programs to lead more healthy, vibrant, fulfilling lives, it is a win-win situation. In fact, more and more employers are incorporating wellness programs, according to a study of 945 companies by Hewitt Associates. The study found that 93 percent of employers currently offer some kind of health promotion program, up from 89 percent in 1996.

Some of the more popular programs include:

- **Health-related education or training**—Seventy-two percent of employers offer employees some kind of education or training, ranging from seminars and workshops to counseling against lifestyle habits that contribute to chronic or acute conditions.
- **Financial incentive and disincentive programs**— Forty-two percent of companies continue to offer incentive programs, the most common being gifts or monetary awards for employees who participate in health appraisals or screenings. Examples of disincentives include charging employees higher medical or life insurance premiums if they smoke or giving a lower medical-benefit payout for not wearing a safety belt while involved in a car accident.
- **Disease management programs**—These programs seek to proactively identify populations who have, or who are at very high risk for, targeted medical conditions. According to the survey, 76 percent of employers currently provide such programs to employees. Eighty-four percent of employers offer these programs through self-insured and/or fully insured health plans.

- **Health risk appraisals**—Twenty-eight percent of employers administer health risk appraisals (questionnaires) to analyze an employee's health history and promote early detection of preventable health conditions. Most employers use appraisals periodically (44 percent) or annually (40 percent).

- **Health screenings**—Screenings are offered by 75 percent of employers, mostly to detect high blood pressure or high cholesterol. Screenings may be offered through health plans, on-site health fairs or mobile units for mammography.

- **Special programs for disease and medical management**—About 79 percent of employers offer flu vaccinations, well baby/child care, and prenatal care.

Source: Hewitt Associates

Chapter Eight

America's Defunct Health-Care System

*The U.S. Government spends $5,035 per person on
health care annually.*

Source: Health Affairs, Jan/Feb 2002

If our health-care system were a patient, it would be dying.

That's right—dying. We'd put it on life support, call in the
minister for last rites and get ready to notify the next of kin that
the patient wouldn't make it through the night. A call to the
local funeral home wouldn't be out of order either. One call we
wouldn't make is to any organ donor program. This patient is
so diseased that nobody would want the organs.

That's not what conventional wisdom—in the form of
uplifting messages from the medical-industrial complex—is
telling us. The pharmaceutical companies, the health-mainte-
nance organizations, and even our own doctors are spending
billions telling us that everything is going to be O.K. "You'll
see," they cry. "Don't you know that we are living in the most
advanced era of modern medicine in human history? So don't
worry about it. Keep eating those cheeseburgers and drinking

those martinis. If you get sick, have we got a prescription drug for you!"

From a business point of view, you can't blame Big Medicine. Billions of dollars have been plowed into the notion that treatment, rather than prevention, is the answer to our health-care problems. There's no money in prevention—at least not as much as there is in treatment—so please don't rock the boat and suggest otherwise. That's the message we're getting from the health-care industry—an industry that from the loftiest CEO to the most humble country doctor has a huge financial stake in seeing that prevention remains out of the spotlight and that treatment reigns supreme.

The way our health system is set up doesn't help either. A combination of conflicting interests—the idea of helping sick people get better, and the idea of producing profits for various levels of the medical-industrial complex that researches, develops, and treats illnesses and disease—all fuel the fire. Other factors are at work that increase the financial burden. "The government's annual bill for health care spending significantly exceeds that of other nations, because physicians' salaries and hospital costs are higher, and medical technology is more widely used," said *The New England Journal of Medicine* (January 7, 1999). "The transfer of funds among federal and state Medicare and Medicaid programs is another important component of national health-care spending. The American health-care system is at once the most expensive and the most inadequate system in the developed world."

The problem is the continuous rise in cost and usage of the health-care system. These rising costs are literally shutting down states. Medicaid—the federal-state health care program for the poor and disabled—now makes up 20 percent of spending by state governments. Medicaid costs fall second only to education, but that may not be the case much longer.

The problem that states face is that they cannot carry a deficit as the federal government is does. Their books have to balance. As I am write this, the states are faced with approximately $68.5 billion in shortfalls. In 2002, Medicaid cost $250 billion, up 13.4 percent from the previous year. This program that was designed to help the poor and disabled get health care is now disabling states and putting them in the poorhouse.

Created by Congress in 1965, Medicaid has reached the point where it pays for one in six Americans. Medicaid pays for one-third of all births, insures almost a quarter of all children, reimburses half the cost of HIV and AIDS treatments and pays for two-thirds of the 1.6 million nursing-home patients. In 2002, enrollment in Medicaid increased an estimated 8.6 percent—the highest increase since 1992—and the program directors are expecting a 7.7 percent increase for 2003. As if that weren't enough, they're also expecting the costs to rise 6 percent.

With such an enormous bill, state governments face the unsavory choice of cutting back. The cuts and potential reductions planned for 2003 represent about 2 percent of the 47 million Americans who receive Medicaid. Two percent doesn't sound like much—but more than one million does and that's how many people we're talking about—one million people without insurance or medical coverage.

In 2003, California is trying to cut 543,000 of the 6.5 million residents receiving Medicaid. And it's not just California. Massachusetts is dropping 44,000; Michigan 52,000; Missouri 20,000; Nebraska 22,532; and Tennessee 160,000. But that may not be enough. In 2002, Nebraska cut the number of people enrolled in Medicaid by 10 percent but still spent 6 percent more on Medicaid that year than the year previous.

According to Jim Tallon, chairman of the Kaiser Commission on Medicaid, states are short on money for Medicaid because rising costs of health care and a recession are making it harder for Americans to pay their bills. And that has many governors concerned. "We simply can't sustain a 10 percent to 15 percent growth continually," said Bob Taft of Ohio.

Inevitably, the cutbacks will mean more people are unable to afford medical care when they need it. That means more sick people getting sicker. Eventually, all those people will begin to roll into the nation's emergency rooms, which by federal mandate must treat everyone who comes in. But what happens when the emergency room becomes the primary care center? Soon people will be turned away from the emergency room—because it will be either full or bankrupt.

As if the price tag weren't already high enough, there are also indirect costs associated with Medicaid and Medicare. Doctors, clinics and hospitals are becoming increasingly frustrated with these programs. Many doctors—frustrated with the rules and low prices paid by Medicare—are beginning to limit the number of Medicare patients they treat while some are refusing to treat any at all, according to a June 2001 USA Today article. Two surveys in Colorado showed that only 15 percent of doctors in that state were accepting new Medicare patients. This same trend was showing up in Georgia, Texas, Washington, and other urban areas. "We're getting more calls from people requesting assistance in finding a physician who will accept Medicare," said Glenda Rogers of the Area Agency in Austin, Tex. "I'm not sure we're in a crisis yet, but we could be in the not-too-distant future."

While the Area Agency may not be in a crisis, those people who reach 65 years of age and are told by their doctors that they have been going to for as long as they can remember that they must now find a new doctor are in crisis. But that's not the only crisis they're facing. Pharmacies are just as frustrated as the doctors.

Because of the high costs and poor economy, many states are cutting back on the amount of money they reimburse for Medicaid. Washington state plans to cut $71 million. Other states that have made or plan to make cuts include Arkansas,

Colorado, Connecticut, Idaho, Illinois, Indiana, Maryland, Mississippi, Montana, Nebraska, North Carolina, Ohio, Oklahoma, South Carolina, and Virginia.

These cuts have pharmacies pitching a fit. "This will send a number of pharmacies over the edge. We're not a religion. We're not here for charity purposes. We've got to make a profit or we can't stay open," said Ernest Boyd, executive director of the Pharmacists Association in Ohio. This has made many pharmacies—including the big chain stores like Rite Aid and Walgreen's—seriously reconsider their involvement in Medicaid. "We believe everyone should have access to medical care," said Karen Rugen, a spokesperson for Rite Aid. "It's just hard to do it below your costs."

"Doctored" Prices

Pharmacies may complain about reductions in Medicaid reimbursement, but just how much can they really say? Look at this example from an April 2003 article in *USA Today*:

A Seattle-based pharmacist would pay his wholesaler $109.76 for a month's supply of Prilosec—a commonly prescribed medicine for stomach problems. Washington Medicaid patients don't pay anything for the Prilosec, but the state would pay $127.35—that's a profit of $17.59. A private insurer would pay $123.61. The reason for the extra $4? Medicaid patients ask more questions and require more paperwork. That may not sound like much money, but consider that the inspector general for the Health and Human Services Department warned states in an August 2003 report that they are overpaying pharmacists by $1 billion a year. Just think of it this way—that extra $4 that pharmacies charge is coming straight out of your paycheck every month.

"Big Brother" may continue to try and step in, but federal involvement in the medical industry is already suffering. When they do try to step in—with Medicare and Medicaid already failing—we will see the practice of rationing reawakened. Many of us weren't around for it, but the World War II years brought with them the trend of "rationing" precious commodities like steel, metal and even chocolate. So too will we see similar rationing of health care over the next ten or twenty years. Countries like Great Britain and Canada, where more socialized health-care systems hold sway, have already begun rationing health care—with disastrous results. More than one million U.K. citizens are on long waiting lists to see physicians for routine matters like checkups. Rationing has also resulted in increased denials in these countries. In the U.K., the number of patients denied treatment includes 9,000 for renal dialysis, 15,000 for cancer chemotherapy, 17,000 for coronary artery surgery, and 7,000 for hip replacement, reported The New York Times. With U.S. health-care costs rising out of control, the health-care industry will have to resort to similar rationing to make ends meet.

Can you hear that long, solid-beep sound? That's the sound of state and federal medical programs flat lining.

HEALTH INSURANCE

Health-insurance premiums are also high and going higher. While more recent numbers aren't readily available, health insurance premiums are most definitely on the rise. According to the Agency for Healthcare Research and Quality (AHRQ), health-insurance premiums rose 30 percent from 1996 to 2000. At roughly 7.5 percent annually, such a rise is double the historic inflation rate of 3.5 percent.

According to the AHRQ, the average annual health insurance premium in 2000 was $2,655 for single coverage and $6,772 for family coverage in private-sector establishments, an increase of 33.3 percent and 36.7 percent respectively since 1996. Other data on health-care cost trends from AHRQ's Medical Expenditure Panel Survey released in November 2002, include:

- Since 1997, the first year that data on retirees was measured, there has been a significant decline in the number of employers who offer health insurance to their retirees of any age. Offerings to retirees under age 65 have dropped from 21.6 percent in 1997 to only 12 percent in 2000. Offerings to retirees 65 and older have dropped from 19.5 percent to 10.7 percent over the same period.

- The proportion of private-sector establishments that offered health insurance rose from 52.9 percent to 59.3 percent between 1996 and 2000. In 2000, almost 90 percent of all employees worked for establishments that offered this coverage, compared with 86.5 percent in 1996.

- Although their employers generally offered health insurance, the portion of private-sector employees actually eligible for coverage fell from 81.3 percent in 1996 to 78.9 percent in 2000. Some employees may not have been eligible, because health insurance was offered only to management or was based on length of service or full-time status. Among those eligible workers, enrollment in plans dropped from 85.5 percent to 81.2 percent over the five years.

Remember, too, that the period between 1996 and 2000 was a period of relative economic growth for Americans. Quite possibly, many businesses and many families could more easily absorb a health-care cost increase that more than doubled the inflation rate. But with the economic gloom of the early 2000's, that argument doesn't hold water anymore.

If health-care costs continue to rise—and the evidence indicates that they will—Americans are headed straight for a health-care crisis the likes of which this country has never seen.

As stated earlier, the costs of dealing with our inattention to good nutritional values alone are spiraling out of control. And despite observations from some corners of our society that good nutritional choices are a "personal" choice, the price we pay for making the wrong diet choices would trigger shock in the most ardent defender of dietary freedom.

Such choices place a burden on all participants in the health-care sector—insurers, customers, and providers.

How so? Any rise in medical costs also takes money out of a health-care provider's budget. That shortfall is made up by the consumer in the form of higher expenses. Plus, "lifestyle" decisions made by individuals that lead to obesity or to ill health (like smoking, drinking, and overeating) hamper society from a financial standpoint because the resulting diseases cause health-care costs to skyrocket for all Americans.

There are other factors that contribute to the incredible rise in costs for health care, including:

- **Technology Breakthroughs**—There's little question that new drugs and surgical treatments have dramatically improved the quality of life for Americans. New technologies that prolong life, like the ones used to provide organ transplants and artificial organs, or technologies used to improve diagnosis, such as Magnetic Resonance Imaging machines, have completely revamped the health-care landscape in a substantially positive way. That said, technology comes at a price. Studies show

that revolutionary new IT innovations comprise roughly 50 percent of the increase in the cost of health care
during the last thirty years.

- **Hefty Insurance Payments**—Older Americans may
  remember the salad days of America's health care, when
  health insurance paid for just about everything and
  when there were no deductibles, co-insurance or co-payment amounts. Today those are only lingering memories. Instead, the health-care industry has shifted to a
  cost-sharing payment platform where consumers pay a
  portion of the cost for the medical care, either in the
  form of co-insurance or a co-payment. Advocates say
  that cost sharing is a big factor in managing health-care
  costs.

- **An Aging Population**—Health-care expenses increase
  when an aging population uses more health-care services
  than a younger one. That's the case in America today,
  especially with seventy-six million Baby Boomers coming down the health-care pipeline.

Conventional wisdom is a funny thing. Even though the
available data shows that we are eating unhealthy foods, leading
stress-ridden lifestyles, and not getting enough exercise,
Americans are nonchalant to such societal factors and the burden they place on our health systems. It's a system that's already
creaking and groaning under the weight of a treatment-first,
prevention-later medicinal mindset.

FACTS:
- In the private sector, companies are increasingly proving less
  and less able to pay for employee health care, according to a
  study conducted by the Henry J. Kaiser Family.

- According to the Foundation and Health Research and Educational Trust, monthly premiums for employer-sponsored health insurance plans jumped 11 percent from spring 2000 to 2001, up from a little more than 8 percent in 2000 and close to 5 percent in 1999. Those numbers jumped to 14 percent in 2002, according to the consulting firm Watson Wyatt, along with a 17 percent jump in the cost of prescription drug benefits. Based on a survey of employers, the Watson Wyatt consulting firm projects an average employer health cost increase of nearly 14 percent nationwide for active employees in 2002. The cost of prescription drug benefits is expected to increase an average of 17 percent next year.

- Long-term care is adding to the cost of health care. Little has been made of it in the media, but Medicaid is now larger than Medicare in terms of the number of people covered—forty-four million vs. forty million, and in totaling spending—$230 billion vs. $215 billion. Medicaid eligibility is also growing twice as fast as Medicare.

- The Institute of Medical News reports that there are roughly forty-one million Americans—about 14.6 percent of the population—without insurance. Worse, in doing so they are reducing everyone's access to health care and even causing job losses. That's because communities with many uninsured residents are more apt to slash hospital services and minimize health prevention and wellness programs. Also, overburdened hospital emergency rooms, required by law to accommodate all comers whether they can pay or not, may be forced to cut services or even shut down.

- A 2002 study by the health advocacy group Families USA, found that nearly 75 million people under age 65 were uninsured for at least one month during 2001 and 2002. Most were from working families, and most were without insurance for at least six months.

- While America's elderly are covered by Medicare, almost one in three people under age 65 went without health insurance at some point during 2001-2002, according to Families USA. Ninety percent of that group was uninsured for at least three months and about 80 percent were from working families.

WE'RE LOSING GROUND

With the cost of health care so prohibitively high, who can say they're surprised when so many Americans can't afford good health care?

One alarming trend resulting from the spiraling costs of health care is that more Americans, including relatively well-off, middle-class Americans, are opting out of paying for health care completely. Yes, the working poor comprise the majority of the 41 million or so Americans who are currently uninsured. But in 2002, the growth rate of working-poor Americans without health care was matched by the growth rate of middle-class Americans who dropped their health-care coverage, because they simply couldn't afford it.

While I understand why out-of-work Americans, home-based and other small business owners, and high-health-risk Americans might want to try and save money by foregoing their health-care plans, the decision to do so is suicidal. Without health care, prohibitive illness or injury could literally bankrupt a family. Worse, they risk not getting the medical care they need when they might need it most.

The decision by Americans affects all of us, too. According to an article in the November 22, 2002 edition of *USA Today*, everybody pays for those who don't have health care—and that raises the cost across the board. "In cases where people can afford insurance but choose not to buy it, they create a societal expense if they go to a public hospital for emergency care, as law mandates that hospitals treat anyone who comes into an emergency room, regardless of their financial situation. Additionally, this reduces the number of healthy people with insurance, which can cause rates to increase overall."

But the picture that such a predicament paints is both heart-rending and eye opening. After all, if middle-class Americans must choose between buying groceries or paying for adequate health care, we have to ask ourselves: What kind of health-care system forces Americans to make that kind of choice?

Not a sustainable one, that's for sure.

Who Is Insured?

According to the Agency for Healthcare Research and Quality (AHRQ), more than 60 percent (seventy-one million) of working Americans under sixty-five years of age have health insurance they obtained through their primary place of employment.

- Among occupational groups, managers and administrators were most likely to be insured (73.3 percent). Farm laborers were least likely to have insurance through their own workplace (28.4 percent).

- Higher hourly earnings were associated with a greater likelihood of workers having health insurance coverage through their primary place of employment. While only one-third of workers making less than minimum wage ($5.15 per hour) had insurance coverage from their primary employer in the first half of 2000, 83.2 percent of workers making more than $21 per hour had insurance.

- Employees who belonged to a labor union were much more likely to be covered by health insurance through their main job than nonunion workers (88 percent of union workers vs. 57.6 percent of nonunion workers).

- Government employees had higher rates of health insurance coverage through their own workplace in 2000 than employees in private industry.

Source: AHRQ Study, February 21, 2003

Chapter Nine

The Responsibility Gap

The year was 1997; I was at a medical conference in New Orleans when my cell phone rang. Barely able to speak, my wife, Michelle, told me her mother Myrna had died. Myrna Jones was a wonderful person and the best grandmother in the world. My daughter, Taylor, loved her so much. Taylor radiated anticipation and excitement when she knew her grandmother was coming over to play. Why did Myrna die? Well, it was simple really: too much food, not enough exercise, and quite possibly the lack of the necessary nutrients to keep her healthy.

A few years later, my daughter's kindergarten class hosted a grandparent's day. In order to make Taylor feel better, we called an elderly friend of ours and ask if she would come serve as a surrogate grandmother. That night during her prayers, Taylor asked God to please take good care of grandma and tell her we miss her. So, what is the cost of being sick? Everything! Exiting this life early will cut your legacy short. I would gladly give up all that I have if it meant my children could enjoy more time with their grandparents.

The next 20 years will be marked by a race to reclaim life and vitality. *The Cost of Being Sick* invites you to take a serious look at your own circumstances and chart a personal course toward a healthier tomorrow. One good turn will lead to another. This remodeling project will ensure greater financial stability, and a legacy marked by fullness of life rather than bouts of lasting sickness. The upside is just that, a climb—an ascent on a path that is less traveled, and one that will undoubtedly make all the difference.

As I said in my adaptation from President Eisenhower's farewell address in the introduction, "Only an alert and knowledgeable citizenry can compel the proper meshing of the huge industrial and medical machinery of treatment with our healthy lifestyles and goals." The balance required to offset the enormous influence of the treatment mentality will demand personal resolve, not federal legislation or corporate compromise. Finding the magic of "Future Charlie" will involve a consistent effort and a starting point.

To conclude, I would like to spend a few moments "meshing" these issues into four easy-to-remember diagrams that will visually model the essentials of *The Cost of Being Sick.*

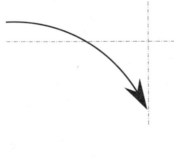

The government's ability to administer Medicare and Medicaid will continue to slip. Corporate America will reduce benefits to boost sagging profits.

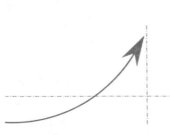

Health-care treatment will continue to outpace inflation by a factor of at least three and quickly become too expensive for the average American to access on demand.

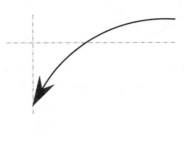

Madison Avenue marketing campaigns, stressed-out work sched-
ules, and our fast-food-eat-on-the-
run culture will continue to grease
the skids for our unhealthy and
sedentary lifestyles.

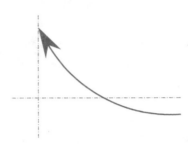

The disease process will grow
increasingly more common with the
aging baby-boom generation; and our
children will start showing symptoms
earlier and with more frequency.

These four diagrams graphically interlock to establish the crux of our dilemma and opportunity. The first quadrant represents the decline in available money to pay for health coverage from both government agencies and the private sector. On the opposite side, our collective lifestyle routines, without any positive changes, will advance the continual degradation of American health. This decline will fuel an upsurge in chronic illness and disease, which will ultimately drive the cost of treatment to unreachable levels for the "citizenry" of America.

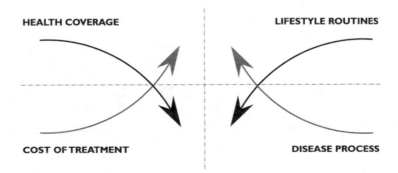

HEALTH COVERAGE   LIFESTYLE ROUTINES

COST OF TREATMENT   DISEASE PROCESS

THE RESPONSIBILITY GAP

Taking action towards prevention rather than relying on treatment will generate two positive outcomes. First, you will protect your lifestyle, meaning the activities that bring you joy and fulfillment, from unwanted ailments. For many, an ideal retirement means playing more golf, spending more time with grandchildren, and taking those road trips with the newly purchased RV. This all works if you and your bottom line are healthy. You cannot bounce your grandchildren on your knee if your body struggles to even support itself. Unfortunately, the current trends indicate that the retirement years for many, perhaps even you, will be marked by fighting for life rather than living it.

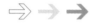

IMPROVED LIFESTYLE PROTECTION

TREATMENT   PREVENTION

Second, moving away from treatment towards prevention will strengthen your financial situation by spending less on the exorbitant cost of health care. Spending $7.50 a month on a multi-vitamin and mineral supplement that bases its strength upon meeting the already flawed RDA benchmark will not cut it. Prevention will cost a little more on the front end. Investing $100 a month as a forty-five year old towards prevention measures will cost you $24,000 by the time you hit the age of sixty-five. According to the study from Fidelity Investments referred to earlier in the book, a couple retiring today at age sixty-five will need approximately $160,000 in savings to cover their retirement medical expenses, assuming that they do not have an employer-sponsored plan. Twenty years from now employer-sponsored health insurance will be the exception, not the rule. Take into consideration that health-care costs continue to rise between 7-15 percent per year and that figure will equal $500,000 to $2,225,000 respectively in twenty years.

The $100 a month investment towards prevention is just as important as any 401(K) contribution. Spending $24,000 to avoid $500,000 in potential medical costs makes good sense. Financial security, even avoiding bankruptcy as a senior, will, for the first time, include a vigilant focus on heath and wellness.

 STRENGTHENED FINANCIAL POSITION

TREATMENT   PREVENTION

My identical twin, Charlie, confronted his physiological health gap by committing to a constructive lifestyle change. The convergence of all four quadrants below produces a similar gap—A Responsibility Gap. You own the fate of the no-man's land found at the axis of this grid. The Responsibility Gap is where two roads will diverge in your life and, I am sorry, you cannot travel both. You must either choose the road of prevention or gamble with the road that is governed by treatment. Better personal lifestyle routines will gradually build a proportional line of defense against unnecessary sickness. Proactive wellness programs sponsored by the private sector will strongly support renewed-personal-health convictions and eventually render the high cost of treatment irrelevant. The Responsibility Gap ultimately starts and ends with you!

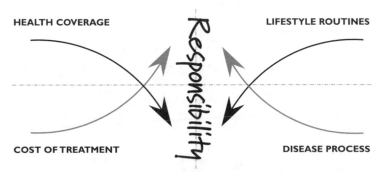

HEALTH COVERAGE   LIFESTYLE ROUTINES

COST OF TREATMENT   DISEASE PROCESS

125

CREATE THE FUTURE YOU

While they are fresh in your mind, I encourage you to revisit some of the thoughts and ideas that surfaced while you read through the past nine chapters. This book was designed as a straightforward, warm-up exercise for a yearlong endeavor. Your mind is limber, and your resolve is purposeful. Take the next few moments and start the process of creating your own success story. Your own "Future Charlie" is within reach!

Dear Future _____,

Today is _____, 20___ and I am resolving to make an investment in you, "Future_____." I commit to you that in one year I will look, feel and live differently. I will make each day a success by living up to the following new healthy habits:

1 _____
_____

2 _____
_____

3 _____
_____

4 _____
_____

I know the journey will not be easy, and when the road turns difficult I resolve to read this letter as a reminder of why I must carry on. I want to provide you a life full of active years and lasting memories.

Signed,

Historical _____

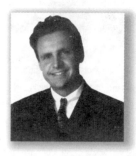

Healthcare Futurist, Nicholas J. Webb has served as the CEO of several medical companies including: Micro Dynamics Medical and SunMedica, Inc. he is one of the founding Partners of Nupak Medical Manufacturing and Talon Medical, additionally he is a Certified Management Consultant and a successful inventor. In fact Nick has just been awarded his twenty-seventh medical product patent from the US Patent and Trademark office.

He is the inventor of the FlexPlug ophthalmic implant, one of the smallest human implants for the treatment of ocular surface disease. His KidMatch product is used by hospitals all over the country to ensure newborns are not switched at birth. He has also invented a wide array of Pharmacology Compliance Devices and micro-surgical instruments.

He and his inventions have been featured on several national television shows, programs including *Nightline NBC, ABC,* and *The Leeza Show.*

Currently, Webb serves as the President of Lassen Scientific, Inc, (www.lassenscientific.com) which specializes in helping organizations to gain a competitive edge by improving employee health and job performance.

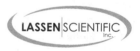

Lassen Scientific, Inc. was founded with the express purpose of applying the latest science and technologies to the area of employee performance and corporate wellness. To learn more about Lassen Scientific log on to our web site at www.lassenscientific.com

LASSEN SCIENTIFIC, INC.

Our strategic mission is to provide the latest technologies in the areas of organizational wellness and employee performance. Our Certified Management Consultants specialize in deploying programs that achieve the highest levels of results and sustainability.

HAPPY HEALTHY HABITS

HAPPY HEALTHY HABITS

Studies suggest that 90 percent of individuals that join sports clubs (Gyms) dropout in just three months. The overwhelming majority of people who endeavor life changing programs fail. Correspondingly the secret to achieving weight loss and other health and lifestyle objectives is not in the tools but rather the development of permanent habits. This powerful program inspires the participant to adopt the five simple steps of permanent habit creation.

This program is available as a keynote, workshop or comprehensive workplace program.

THE COST OF BEING SICK

This powerful program accurately communicates the future of healthcare in America. Moreover this program provides the participant a roadmap on how to prepare and protect their family against these emerging trends. Some of the predictions include:

- Why most Americans will never be able to retire.
- How healthcare cost will replace the mortgage payment as a family's biggest monthly expense.
- How a well-defined National Health Score will affect all aspects of their lives.
- How wellness programs will protect individuals both physically and financially.

This program is available as a keynote, workshop or comprehensive workplace program.

FUTURE CHARLIE

Wouldn't it be great if you could simply set down an architect the perfect future you? This unique program follows the case study of "Future Charlie." This powerful program provides a step-by-step process on goal setting that gets results every time.

This program is available as a keynote, workshop or comprehensive workplace program.

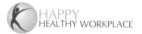

HAPPY HEALTHY WORKPLACE

This comprehensive program provides the ultimate solution for the modern workplace. This program includes on-site consulting, training and facilitation with the simple objectives of significantly improving employee productivity and health. This powerful program addresses all aspects of employee health and productivity including:

- Stress management
- Weight management
- Conflict resolution
- Employee performance
- Quality of work life
- Participation compliance
- Compensation and Decompensation programs

Through our strategic partners Lassen Scientific Inc. can provide a turnkey solution for all aspects of employee performance and corporate wellness.

This program is available as a keynote, workshop or comprehensive workplace program.

HAPPY HEALTHY COMMUTER

Without question the single biggest pitfall in the deployment of a wellness and quality of work life initiative is compliance. Human behavioral experts know that the repetition of a powerful message is fundamental to driving permanent compliance. The *Happy Healthy commuter* is an entertaining monthly audiotape program that is created in a talk show format. This program keeps your employees on track providing you a sustainable employee initiative.